Feel Well, *Play* Well

Amazing Golf
through
Whole Health

Dr. Gil Winkelman, ND, MA

Contents

To my father Peter, for teaching me to play the game of golf and my son Eli who reminded me that it was fun to play.

Preface to this Edition

Much has changed since the first edition of this book hit Amazon. For me personally, my life and practice transformed. I practice at a different clinic than I did splitting my time between Hawaii and Portland. I've also written a novel that should be out around the time of this edition coming out.

But my approach to health hasn't changed that much.I still recommend yoga. I suggest dietary changes for many patients. I recommend meditation, mindfulness, or some other breathing practice to all who see me. But some things are very different. I focus more on the Walsh Protocol or nutrient therapy. (see http://askdrgil.com/walsh-protocol for more information.)

Why am I doing that? It gets results. Though Dr. Walsh designed the protocols around treatment of mental illness I've found it to help athletes of all kinds. And why wouldn't it? Balancing the body helps improve our mental function. Most Americans are zinc deficient, a problem that affects every system in the body including, immunity, the musculoskeletal system, the brain, and digestion. Most importantly, it helps almost 75-80% of my patients with anxiety, thought issues, learning problems, concentration issues, and depression without other interventions. Simply taking vitamins helps you feel better!

I hope you enjoy this book and find it helpful.

In health,
Dr. Gil

Introduction

What Does Holistic Health Have to do with Amazing Golf?

Simple chance created the *Feel Well, Play Well* program. When I started in private practice, I wasn't treating golfers; I treated mostly people with concussions including surfers, and football, basketball, and hockey players. My expertise was traumatic brain injury. I had great success using holistic medicine and neurofeedback to help people overcome anxiety, insomnia, weight gain, headaches, and learning difficulties. All of those symptoms are problems that arise due to head trauma.

Golfers generally do not receive head trauma. But many people including executives, business owners, and other golfers have issues with the symptoms mentioned above. A patient whom I'll call Jim had received multiple small head traumas in his line of work as a construction worker. He tended to work underneath houses and would often bang his head. Like many of the people I worked with who had head traumas, Jim had memory issues, focus and concentration problems, numbness and tingling in his hands and feet, and trouble sleeping. Some people have other issues after head injury including headaches, weight gain, and digestive issues, but Jim had avoided those. He came to me, though, not for his golf game but because his wife dragged him to my office. According to her, Jim had attention issues, wasn't a good listener, had trouble sleeping, and was falling behind at work

I had been working with Jim for several weeks, when one week he came for his weekly appointment and said that nothing was different. I was skeptical. The stress lines on his face were gone, his eyes had a different quality to them such that he had better focus, his ability to answer my questions was more specific and coherent, and he spoke without hesitation and knew exactly what I was asking. I pressed him further.

"Is your concentration better?" I asked.

"Well one thing I have noticed is that my golf game is improving," he said.

"How so?" I asked.

"I am shooting about five strokes better than I had been and I broke 80 for the first time in my life. Could that be related to what we are doing here? "

Jim was in his 60s and was a consistent golfer. He generally shot in the mid-80s occasionally going over 90.

"Why do you think you are scoring better?" I asked.

"I don't know how to describe it but my mind seems quieter when I'm playing. I am able to think about my shots better. Also, the aches and pains in my hands and feet are gone."

"Are you sleeping better, too?"

"Come to think of it, yes I am," he responded. "I guess all of those things are helping my game."

When his wife came to the next appointment, she told me he was doing better at work and at home. He was more attentive and able to remember things again.

The *Feel Well, Play Well* program came out of this and other similar interactions as I realized that there were many things that could be done to help golfers. As a Naturopathic Physician (see below as to what a N.D. is licensed to do) I mostly treat neurological problems and physical problems that interface with the brain in some manner. My training includes a BA in Genetics from UC Berkeley, an MA in Counseling Psychology, and five years of medical school. I have managed to combine all three in my work as a physician as I investigate people's genetic make-up to understand their health situation and use my counseling skills to assess and help their mental and emotional states. Many of the conditions I treat require a good understanding of these three aspects in order to affect real change in the health and well-being of our patients.

Head trauma is one thing that I treat, but often people come to me without knowing they've had an injury or that the injury is related to their symptoms. I treat people with autism, anxiety, insomnia, neurological deficits, fatigue, obsessive-compulsive disorder, depression, migraine headaches, high blood pressure, digestive ailments, asthma, and many other conditions.

Many people find us because of our experience with treatment of post-concussion syndrome and its associated symptoms such as anxiety, insomnia, depression, weight gain, attention deficit issues, and other ailments. Many of these people are golfers who, like Jim, started reporting improvements in their game. They report having fewer injuries, less pain while playing, and scoring better as well. What I discovered was that a combination of nutrition, exercise, neurofeedback, botanical remedies, meditation, and breathing techniques could make someone a better golfer. The *Feel Well, Play Well* program was born!

Who Does It Help?

Many of these people are busy executives and small business owners that want to get better at golf but don't necessarily have time to practice more often. The *Feel Well, Play Well* program allows them to improve their golf game while working on their health issues. And it helps them to succeed better in business too. According to a study from Europe, on average executives that play golf well earn 17% more than those who do not play well or do not play at all. Creating better health, a better game, and making more money — what other reasons do you need to continue reading?

The program helps people improve their game while improving their health. Increased health means better sleep, more energy, stable moods, fewer injuries, and better concentration. Many patients come to us because they have chronic problems that haven't improved with conventional treatments. Some people's condition is such that they cannot play golf when they start with us; their injuries are too severe to play the game. This book can help people begin the recovery process. This book is mostly focused, however, on helping people to improve their game while improving their health.

For the person who is currently in good health, the exercises and techniques in the book provide you with tools to maintain health as you grow older. As we age, we lose strength, balance, and flexibility if we don't take care of ourselves. It is sad to see people who have worked so hard their entire lives to have money for retirement to not be able to enjoy it due to health problems. While I have had success helping older adults gain function back, it is much harder than if you maintain flexibility, strength, and balance when you are younger.

At the end of the book, I describe what I do in my practice. But most of health begins with you. There are aspects of this program that can be done at home by anyone. What does nutrition, exercise, meditation, breathing, and relaxation (or better sleep) equal? These are the five principles of yoga. And all of these are things that I give patients to do away from the clinic, and I realized that all of this information could be shared in a book format.

This book is a beginning. It is an opportunity for someone to use the ideas and techniques to improve one's golf game and avoid injuries in the process. However, it is much more than that. These techniques help one live a fuller life. How can I say that? Because even if your game doesn't improve, you will experience greater enjoyment of the game and your life will improve. And why play a game if it's not fun? Read on and learn how to improve your health and your game.

What is a Naturopath?

The term Naturopath means different things in different places. For many years it was synonymous with what we would now call a medical doctor. In many states in America, a Naturopath is similar to a nutritionist. They provide dietary advice, recommend supplements, and may also be trained in herbal medicine. In Oregon, Washington, California, Arizona, and ten other states, a Naturopathic Physician or ND, is a type of physician similar to a Medical Doctor or Osteopathic Doctor. We are trained as primary care physicians that can prescribe pharmaceuticals, perform physical exams, order labs, and do minor surgery. In some of those states, including Oregon, we are licensed to perform physical adjustments similar to chiropractors. While the scope of practice between NDs, MDs and DOs is similar, the focus is very different. As a general rule, NDs are trained to take a holistic view of the body. This means that an ND's training requires them to look at how different parts of the body affect other parts. This provides a huge advantage in diagnosing a patient, but more importantly, it allows for proper treatment. (Obviously there are MDs and DOs who are very holistic, but their training at medical school often is not.)

Yoga: A Healthy Lifestyle Choice

Many of our patients ask what types of exercises are good for them and why do them. The short answer is anything that makes you feel good. For many people just walking regularly is enough, but others don't find that stimulating; they want something that will build strength, cardiovascular tone, and flexibility. Yoga is perfect for all three. Yoga as an exercise allows for movement that stretches and strengthens the body. While there are different forms, generally it involves doing poses that are held for a certain amount of time and done in sequence. The sequence can be important but allows for you to do them in a flowing motion that can assist in heart health.

I have experienced profound changes due to yoga on a personal level. I spent years not doing any sort of deep stretching exercises. Besides playing golf, I also played ice hockey, only performing minimal stretches at the rink or stretching before or after weight training. That was until the day my back seized up on the ice. I could barely get the equipment off myself because I was in so much pain. I was unable to walk or move for about ten days, and I couldn't play hockey for about four months. I took various sorts of supplements, herbal remedies, and had bodywork to help release the tight spots in my body. Between my rehab visits to my healthcare providers, I started stretching. As I opened up the tissue spaces and released toxins, I gained greater flexibility. I started to move in ways that I could not previously. I did yoga more often and for longer sessions, until one day I found myself able to get into positions I had not been in since high school. I wasn't supposed to be lifting heavy weights, so I was not going to the gym at all, but after some time I gained muscle mass, looking leaner, and more toned. Eventually I went back to the ice and found I could still keep up. I hadn't lost as much in the way of cardiovascular tone as I thought I would have. I found that my chance of injury was reduced because I am less likely to strain muscles. This convinced me that yoga was an excellent regime and I continue to do it to this day.

Yoga provides an opportunity to build flexibility and strength in a safe manner, but yoga is much more than that. It is a system that releases toxins from the body; toxins that may endanger the body to further injury.

Golf in particular carries risk of injury due to the one-way nature of the sport. What I mean is that the focus of the swing is primarily in one direction. The back swing creates a repetitive strain on that side and can create problems in the lower back. This sort of repetitive strain increases the risk for injury. The number one reason for chronic golf injuries is inadequate warm-ups. Approximately 45% of golfers have chronic injuries, and of those, the majority are due to a lack of flexibility or poor conditioning. Yoga helps minimize this risk, as we will see. It also allows a person to strengthen the opposing muscles groups that do not get used while playing golf. Yoga can help prevent these injuries, but also relieve and reduce the chronic nature of injuries as well.

The focus of this book is golf. Not only do we want to use yoga to protect your body from injury, but we want to give you exercises that will improve your game. Many professional athletes have turned to yoga to improve their game. Golfers, hockey players, football players, and others are using yoga to improve their health and help injuries. NHL players who perform yoga regularly claim that they require fewer repetitions of weights to gain greater strength and remain flexible.

Yoga also helps quiet the mind. When the mind is quiet, it is easier for the body to perform difficult tasks. That quiet allows muscle memory to take over so that the ball can be struck properly. Overall, we are finding that people who practice yoga score better. Some patients find they hit the ball farther, while others do not. All of them enjoy themselves much more.

Yoga encompasses more than just a bunch of exercises; it also includes meditation, diet, relaxation, and breathing. All of these topics will be discussed in the context of golf and how each can be used to improve one's score.

Each pose will be described, its benefits discussed, and where it might be felt in the body. Some people will not be able to do every pose. The goal is to work towards all of them as closely as possible. If you are finding that doing a pose causes pain in places not described in the photo, stop the pose. It is probably time to seek professional help in that situation, as you could have a more serious health concern such as a torn ligament or tendon, nerve impingement, or a slipped vertebral disk. Later in the book, types of pain will be discussed. Understanding different types of pain is important, as some pain can be good because it is the body stretching itself.

The Five Principles of Yoga

Yoga is a spiritual practice that has principles as a foundation. These principles may be important for some people to manifest the greatest improvements to their game. There are many different approaches and beliefs about yoga, but generally there are five principles agreed upon as the basis for yoga. These principles are very important to an athlete and include exercise, breathing, relaxation, nutrition, and meditation. The poses are the exercise and breathing portion of this, but they are by no means the only portion. All of these aspects go together and integrate together. A healthy diet, for example, allows the body to relax and breathe more easily. When one is unable to relax, one cannot meditate or breathe properly. Below is a brief description of each of the principles. Each section of the book will cover one of these principles.

1. Nutrition: Otherwise known as Diet

Nutrition may be one of the most important aspects of health and yoga. As the saying goes, "you are what you eat." Modern science has attempted to distill food down to its core components: carbohydrates, fats, proteins, and calories. If you eat the right combination of each, and don't eat others, then you will be healthy. It also assumes that if you burn more calories than you take in, you won't gain weight. In my practice neither of these assumptions are entirely accurate. I don't think too many people would believe that eating a Twinkie is the same as eating the same caloric intake of kale. Kale provides nutrients and minerals not found in Twinkies and some argue is more easily recognized by the body. Foods that are processed do not have the same nutrient value as foods found in the nature. For that reason, the caloric equation isn't exactly true either. I have seen many patients who only ate one meal a day that was fast food and couldn't understand why they were gaining weight when they were exercising and otherwise taking care of themselves. The right foods at the right times and in the right amounts allow the body to operate at its highest level. Furthermore, one extremely important aspect of diet is hydration, a topic that will be covered in great detail. Understanding the importance of diet is one factor in improving your play.

2. Breathing

Breathing is vital to proper yoga technique. This requires rhythmic breathing and full utilization of lung muscles to absorb oxygen and release toxic waste. Proper breathing provides sufficient utilization of the food that we eat through improved oxygen usage. This provides more energy throughout the day. Breathing can be extremely useful in a sporting event particularly golf. Through it, one may regain composure and be able to salvage a bad hole. We will discuss these concepts further to learn how to use techniques to control emotions better.

3. Relaxation

Breathing and exercise and very important to proper relaxation. Relaxation is vital to help one de-stress. Our modern world is extremely stressful on a regular basis. Relaxation is important to revitalizing the nervous system, regenerating sore muscles and finding an inner sense of peace. One of the most important relaxation exercises we do is sleep. Improper sleep patterns and sleep disturbances can affect our game more than we realize. Poor sleep prevents injuries from healing, can lead to memory and concentration impairment, and affect one's mood. We will discuss more about these problems and how to identify the mechanism leading to the sleep disturbances.

4. Meditation

Meditation is one of the pillars of Yoga and of a great golf game. Many people have a hard time with the idea of meditation. There's something foreign about it for Westerners. But it is crucial not only to golf but to success in life in general. Meditation is a way to gain control over your mind. In yoga beliefs, the mind controls the body and the breath and therefore is key to gaining top physical and mental well-being. When one can control one's mind, it allows for improved performance. Starting with just a few minutes a day you too can experience the benefits of a quiet mind.

5. Exercise

Exercise is what most people think of when they think about yoga. It is called Hatha Yoga, which refers to a series of poses that can be used to lead to the purification of the body and the mind to provide for more vital energy. In yoga philosophy, the body is viewed as a temple. Better spiritual and mental health begins with improved physical health. Recent studies suggest that one is more likely to become ill when one views the body and mind as separate entities. One neglects caring for oneself and neglects exercise, proper diet, and relaxation.

The benefit of doing the exercise sequences or asanas is that you gain strength and flexibility while relieving tightness and joint pain. The poses range from the simple, such as standing at attention, to holding yourself up with one arm. Each pose was selected to assist someone who plays golf. The poses can be done quickly or can be stretched over a longer time period. The second half of the book pertains to these exercises.

Having reviewed the five principles, let's discuss each one in more depth. The importance of each to a golfer will be discussed in the context of how the body works. Then at the end, we will put this all together when we discuss what we do at our clinic. With that, let's dive into the yoga principles and learn the tips for health and improving your game.

Chapter 1

Eat Well, Play Well: What you Eat and Drink Affects Your Score

When I started practicing medicine, many of my patients believed that my goal was to give them dietary advice. They would want to know what to eat to lose weight, feel better, improve sleep or mood, and so forth. Of course, I would give some ideas about what to eat to help with a particular issue. As I began to know the patient better, I would give more and more specific advice. Generally, I started simple because most patients weren't ready to make radical changes all at once. But each little change added up and over time, my patient's diet and health improved.

Nutrition refers to intake of sustenance into the body, including food and water. A balanced diet is important for anybody, but it is extremely important for athletes. Just like one wouldn't put cheap gas in a high-performance car, one shouldn't eat junk food and expect to perform well long-term.

Over time I learned that though what you put in your body is very important, what comes out of your body is also important. Not only does what you eat fuel your body appropriately, but understanding some of the principles of food, water, and toxicity can help one's performance and reduce possible injury. Many injuries are exacerbated by high levels of inflammation in the body. Reducing inflammation not only reduces the risk and severity of injury, but it can also help prevent other ailments such as heart disease, cancer, and stroke. Let's start our exploration of nutrition by discussing toxicity and elimination. By exploring how toxicity can build up in the body and the ways to better eliminate those toxins, we can better understand why diet is so important.

Ways to Help Physical Pain: Releasing Toxins

Imagine a bucket where the bucket keeps filling with water and over time starts to get more and more full. At the bottom is a release valve that allows water to leave the bucket. If the valve is not clogged and the rate of flow of water into the bucket is slow, the bucket will not overflow. If, however, the valve becomes clogged or the flow of water into the bucket increases, the valve can't keep up and the bucket will overflow. Our bodies are like that bucket and the water is like toxins.

The body-as-a-bucket analogy is an important construct to better understand why diet and nutrition is so important to toxicity in the body. Toxins come from a variety of places. The body produces some, as they are the waste products of digestion and metabolism. Others come from our environment. We breathe them in the air, eat them in our food, and sometimes absorb them through our skin. Golf courses can have high levels of toxicity due to the chemicals used to keep the courses beautiful. (For example, never put a tee in your mouth because of the high levels of fertilizers and pesticides used on a golf course.) We eliminate these toxins through our kidneys as we urinate, our digestion through defecation, and our lungs by breathing. When those three systems don't work well, we start to eliminate toxins through our skin, or we might not release the toxicity at all and store them in fat cells, joint spaces, or in our nervous system. This can lead to weight gain, joint pain, muscle pain, and/or problems with the nervous system.

Let's say you eat a cheeseburger from a fast food place filled with chemicals, pesticides, hormones, and antibiotics. The meat, while natural, comes from cows that ate pesticide-sprayed grain, were injected with growth hormones, and then given antibiotics due to the close living quarters. The meat is 30% fat. The bun is filled with chemical preservatives, wheat that was processed to have no nutrients and sprayed with pesticides. The condiments are full of high fructose corn syrup and the cheese isn't real. None of these things by themselves is harmful. One could eat this every once in a while and not suffer any ill effects other than some indigestion. But all of this creates a load on the body. It requires the body to work harder to eliminate toxicity. Even if you were to eat kale that had pesticides on it, your body would need to work to eliminate toxins. This is the basis for dietary changes. With fewer toxins in our system, the body can maintain effective elimination, thereby decreasing the risk of disease and injury.

Another important component of eliminating toxins is consuming foods that can be broken down so that nutrients can be absorbed and also leave some non-soluble materials to leave as excrement. Most of us have been told to eat fiber. Non-soluble fiber can absorb toxins in the body, and since it's not readily digestible, it is easily eliminated. (Soluble fiber, by contrast, is absorbable on some level but mainly helps to absorb cholesterol and increases fullness during a meal.)

The liver works at removing toxins by filtering the blood and moving the toxins into the digestive system for removal. If there is a delay in removing the toxins, they could migrate back into the body because of the delay. This could defeat the purpose of the liver's function. Regular bowel habits are very important for this reason, which is why eating fruits and vegetables with soluble and insoluble fiber is so important. Ensuring that all the elimination pathways are available is important, but nothing compares to drinking water.

> **Tip:** If you are not getting your 25–50 grams of fiber per day, increase that amount slowly over the course of 3–6 weeks. An increase in fiber can lead to problems of gas and bloating.

Drink Water!

Probably the most important and under-utilized dietary necessity is drinking water. Although our bodies are comprised mostly of this substance (70% by weight), water is an essential nutrient because we lack the capacity to produce it in the required amounts. An astonishing amount of water—70,000 liters—diffuses through our blood vessels every day, transporting nutrients and removing metabolic wastes and toxins that have accumulated around cells. Pure water is the only substance that can accomplish these awesome processes that are necessary for our continued health and wellness. Furthermore, without enough water, the kidneys cannot function optimally. As a result, the liver compensates, which can detract from its ability to eliminate other toxins from the bloodstream.

The body depends on a state of adequate hydration to complete many of its essential physiological processes.

Many chemical reactions are water dependent including the processes that our body uses to create energy.

Proteins and enzymes function more efficiently with water, so the body's ability to heal depends on sufficient amounts of water. Without these processes being efficient, one's ability to recover from injury is impaired and muscles won't perform to optimal levels. Furthermore, neurological function is profoundly impacted by an individual's state of hydration.

The brain is 85% water when the body is hydrated; in a state of dehydration, neurological function is hindered. The affected functions make sense when we consider the responsibilities of the various parts of the brain. The limbic system, which is below the cortex, completes emotional processing and primitive survival urges. The reptilian brain governs basic functions in the body such as breathing and heart rate. The cortex is responsible for motor functions and thought and is the outer layer of the brain. During dehydration, the body must prioritize which areas of the brain will receive the water that is available; the survival-oriented reptilian brain is less likely to become dehydrated than the information-oriented cortex. The resulting cognitive impairments may mirror this prioritization: when the brain is not adequately hydrated, we decrease cortical functions of abstract thinking and concentration. We also may be more likely to respond more emotionally as opposed to rationally and be less equipped to handle stress. Moreover, a glass of water is one-third oxygen, and this fact alone has implications for the ability of water to contribute to optimal brain function.

Think about how this might affect your round of golf if you are dehydrated. Your heart rate may rise, your body becomes more stressed, and your ability to think through a shot becomes impaired. Even if you hit the ball well, it may not be in the right direction or aligned with the needs of that particular shot. And if you hit a poor shot, your ability to recover is diminished. With a high enough level of dehydration, your ability to use your muscles becomes impaired and even a slight drop in performance can affect outcomes in golf.

Additional physiological functions of water include the following:

- Water incorporates into proteins and glycogen, playing a structural role.

- Regulation of body temperature from the skin requires water, and so does a youthful appearance and elasticity of skin.

- Water improves gland and hormone function.

- Water is used by the liver to catabolize and liberate fat.

- Water carries nutrients, minerals, vitamins, proteins hormones, and chemical messengers.

- Water lubricates and releases wastes and toxins from cells.

- Mental performance, arithmetic ability, short-term memory, and visuomotor tracking are decreased with just a 2% deficit in bodily fluid!

- Studies on athletes have found that a 2% loss of water negatively affects both physical and mental performance by 20%. A 2012 study published in the Journal of Strength and Conditioning Research revealed that even mild dehydration can impair distance, accuracy and distance judgment in golfers.

Water is lost through skin, lungs, urine, and stool on a daily basis. These fluids must be replaced. Not accounting for the loss due to perspiration, 4% of total body weight is the daily turnover of water in adults (15% in infants). Dehydration is gradual and rarely overtly noticed. We lose our sense of thirst as we age, and even then, the signal of thirst happens only after we are already lacking adequate amounts of water. Caffeinated beverages and alcohol, as well as an arid environment, are factors that can decrease hydration. For each cup of alcoholic or caffeinated beverages consumed, two additional cups of water should be consumed beyond the suggestions based on weight. Recognize that the stress response generated by inadequate water intake becomes habitual and we gradually become accustomed to the excess cortisol release; readjusting our physiology to the state of lesser stress takes time and may feel unfamiliar at first.

> **Tip:** You want to be drinking about half your weight in ounces of water. (Check with your doctor if you have any sort of kidney or endocrine disease.) Most people find that if they don't drink that much water, they are going to the bathroom all of the time to compensate for this amount. Drink ½ cup of water every ½ hour. Try not to drink too much water prior to bedtime, as that will cause waking in the middle of the night. Once you begin drinking close to the proper amount you will find that you want to drink that much water and it won't seem like too much.

During a round of golf it is essential to stay hydrated, as the air and heat are sapping your body of moisture at accelerated rates. Most people consume non-hydrating beverages during a round of golf such as an alcoholic or caffeinated beverage. If you don't care about your score or how your feel, it probably doesn't matter to you (and you wouldn't be reading this book!). When it is hot especially, people lag behind in terms of their ability to think, concentrate, and their amount of energy. By hydrating, you will have more muscle power, energy, and mental clarity as you get into the last six holes of a round. If you sweat a lot, even more water is required.

(Side Note: Sports drinks such as Gatorade are extremely popular and highly advertised. For most people, they are also unnecessary. Unless you are playing a round of rapid golf whereby you do full sprints between shots, water should be sufficient for hydration.)

> **Tip:** Many older golfers have prostate and/or gout issues. These often start due to kidney imbalance and one can lead to the other as prostate difficulties makes one not want to use the bathroom. If you are experiencing urination issues or you have a history of gout or other types of stones, see your doctor about appropriate treatment.

The Focus on Diet or the Diet of Focus?

While there is much focus on diet in the media, there is less attention given to how diet can affect your concentration. Diet can impact mood, concentration, and mental health greatly. In my practice I see many people with a large variety of what may be termed mental health issues. These can include depression, anxiety, and attention deficit disorder. Many times I treat these with dietary changes alone. Why is this important to a golfer? What you eat could be affecting various aspects of your game including muscle strength, heart rate and your ability to focus.

Several studies have shown that various changes in diet can affect one's ability to perform properly. If a certain food affects your heart rate, for example, you will be less able to hit the ball well. But it is the diet's affect on mood and focus that is most curious. Removal of foods by many of my patients has lead to profound relief in concentration problems, sleep problems, anxiety and depression. Artificial colors in particular can be detrimental to your mood, focus, and overall performance. Each person is unique in that different foods will affect everyone differently. Professional assistance can often help one identify problem foods and find alternatives.

Supplementation with appropriate vitamins and minerals can help too. Generally, I do not recommend a multivitamin due to fact that many of the items in the vitamin don't absorb well together. For example, calcium and zinc will interact with one another if taken at the same time. We customize vitamins for our individual patients, but we also have general packages geared towards particular issues such as sleep problems, fatigue, and concentration difficulties. Each are formulated to assist with general health.

So What Should You Eat?

If diet can affect our focus, concentration, mood, and performance, what should we eat? Our clinic offers extremely detailed and individualized nutritional advice. In this book, it is challenging to offer any specific suggestions, as it is not clear what challenges and needs each individual reader will face. Everybody has slightly different needs. They have problems that have arisen due to past food choices, injuries, levels of inflammation, and food sensitivities. I have even seen twin brothers with differences in food sensitivities that required different diets.

There are some important guidelines that we can provide in terms of how to eat.

- Don't eat a big meal prior to playing a round of golf. Players will often eat something large (and maybe fatty) on a hot day before playing. This has the effect of making you fatigued, particularly on hot days.

- Eat whole foods. Whole foods have more nutrients than processed foods and generally provide for better digestion as well.

- Eat plenty of fiber. Between 25–35 grams is required for the average adult.

- Ensure that you have something healthy on hand to eat if you feel your energy dipping during a round. If you are walking the course, you are more likely to get hungry than if you used a golf cart. Mental work also uses energy. Be sure you are properly fueled. One common food that people bring during a round of golf is a banana. They are an excellent food filled with vitamins, minerals, and just the right amount of calories.

- Eat slowly and chew your food. The term "Fletcherize" refers to chewing each bite 32 times to make sure that everything is completely broken down prior to swallowing. Not only does this make digestion easier for the body, but it also means that you are less likely to overeat. Increased production of acid through the act of chewing also means that digestion is more complete.

- Eat at the right times. There are many debates
  about how many meals to eat, how often to eat,
  is it best to eat breakfast, and so forth. The short
  answer is that everyone is different. But one rule
  everyone should follow is to not eat within three
  hours of going to bed. This is because one needs
  time to digest their food and the body needs appropriate fuel to repair the body during sleep. If
  not given enough time, the body will not be able
  to convert this food into proper stores that can be
  utilized. And if one doesn't eat enough, one may
  awaken due to hunger too early in the morning.
  This will be discussed in more detail in the chapter on relaxation.

- Pay attention to foods that may affect you ad-
  versely. Several golfers, including Michelle Wie,
  have eliminated gluten to help improve athletic performance. Different athletes have different reasons for this, including clearing brain
  fog, reducing joint paint, and helping insomnia.
  Gluten is only one of many different foods that
  might cause a reaction. It might be necessary to
  keep a diet dairy to assist you when looking for
  reactions. Make sure that you pay attention to
  the symptoms to see if there are patterns, which
  could happen even two days after the food was
  consumed.

Chapter Summary

- Toxins can accumulate in the body that can create pain and lead to injury. Proper elimination is important for prevention of these problems.

- Drinking enough water is critical to performance. Without enough water, our mental and physical performance can drop without us realizing the cause.

- Proper supplementation can be important to solving various physical problems that arise in your life. Supplementation can help with sleep, mental clarity, injury prevention, and wound healing. Consulting with a healthcare professional can be immensely helpful when selecting supplements.

- Get professional nutritional advice. Knowing specifically what can help you individually is key to proper performance and health.

Chapter 2

Breathing: The Foundation of a Good Golf Swing

Patients will often ask me if I lose my cool on the golf course. They see me as a mild mannered fellow who laughs and has fun while working; some even say that they can't imagine that I get upset after a bad shot. In reality, I do get upset and sometimes I show it by slamming a club into my bag. Generally, though, I just breathe through it and move on.

Breathing is necessary for life. Breathing provides oxygen to cells in our body so that it can function optimally, heal injuries, and energize muscles. It is also important for calming the mind in stressful situations. Without proper levels of oxygen, our body performs at sub-optimal levels.

But how many people discuss the importance of breathing in golf? Golfers need to have proper breathing techniques to optimize performance. There are several reasons for this, including the emotional benefits of proper breathing

to how breathing affects your nervous system and physiology. Not only can proper breathing improve focus, it
can add yardage to your shots. Before giving exercises on
how to improve breathing, let's explore the reasons why
breathing is so important.

When I started doing research for this book I stumbled
upon tidbits about Bobby Jones using breathing to help
his concentration. Jones was arguably one of the greatest
golfers ever. He understood the importance of breath for
calming the mind, keeping the swing in rhythm and staying focused.

Breathing affects various states in our body, especially our
emotions. Shallow breathing sends signals to the brain that
there is danger stimulating the sympathetic nervous system. The sympathetic nervous system takes over and generates more biochemicals that put us into a fight or flight
response. With proper breathing the parasympathetic nervous system (relaxation) takes over. This creates a more
relaxed state and improves concentration. (A discussion
about the parasympathetic and sympathetic nervous systems is in the next chapter.)

Improper breathing can also create problems. Carbon di-
oxide or CO_2 is a waste product of cell function in humans.
When we breathe, we take in oxygen and remove CO_2.
Without proper breathing, there is too much CO_2 in the
blood stream and that can cause the body to not release
enough oxygen into the blood stream. In a state of hyper-
ventilation, for example, the body will be in a vicious cycle
of rapid breathing that leads to panic, and panic leads to
rapid breathing. CO_2 levels increase leading to oxygen being more tightly bound to red blood cells. This can cause
spasms, increase pain and blood pressure, and interfere
with proper neural functioning.

Finally, if breathing is too shallow or if one is winded prior to taking a shot, one is more likely to make a mistake. That's because when we leave our optimal functioning zone of heart rate and breathing, we lose muscle control and focus. There have been several studies on this subject, including Dr. Neil Wolkodoff's work, which showed that golfers slightly out of breath were much more likely to miss a shot than if they were not out of breath. Bobby Jones understood this and admitted that he was trying to catch his breathe at times he pretended to be reading where to hit the ball.

To help with becoming winded easily, some form of cardiovascular exercise is important to one's golf game. While there is a separate chapter on exercise, cardiovascular exercise is a prime component of golf conditions. Even if you ride in a cart when you play (which I do not recommend), you will at times have to walk up a steep incline prior to hitting the ball, and you could become winded. Breathing and cardiovascular conditioning can help with your recovery time so this doesn't occur. Physical fitness is part of that equation, but breathing properly can help improve your endurance.

Would you be willing to walk if you could score better? Dr. Wolkodoff's research showed something else that was intriguing. Walking a course allowed one to score better than riding in a cart. Golfers who had a caddie or pushed their clubs scored better than golfers who rode in a cart or who carried their own bags. Most people I play with feel they have a better feel for the course when walking. The caddie part of this equation may be skewed from the standpoint that a caddie knows the course and can give advice as to club selection. It's also nice to not have to think about your bag and just be handed the club you need when you need it.

Walkers definitely burn more calories than golfers that ride in a cart. Dr. Wolkodoff found that golfers who walked (regardless of having a caddie, a push cart or carrying their clubs) burned about 700 calories per 9 holes while a rider only burned 411 calories under the same conditions. As far as a whole health choice, walking is preferred if you can do so.

Doesn't Everyone Breathe Properly?

What does proper breathing mean? Proper breathing allows for full range of motion of the lungs and ribcage for maximum airflow. In other words, one must be able to inhale and exhale fully. Consistent breathing is very important in golf for the reasons stated previously, and also gives one something to focus on other than the difficulty of the shot. This provides a calming step prior to the shot and creates a routine.

Most people breathe with their chests but it actually starts in the belly. Breathing through the nose is more beneficial as the nasal cavities are designed to provide optimal temperature of air prior to entering the lungs. Breathing from the belly isn't really what you are doing but rather expanding your diaphragm. The diaphragm is a thin muscle at the bottom of the lungs that acts as a bellows when used properly to expand and contract the lungs. This allows for them to be filled and emptied completely. We use the small muscles between our ribs called intercostals that allow for the ribcage to completely expand and contract with the movement of the lungs.

As a side note, posture is extremely important for breathing. When the back is hunched over the diaphragm cannot move properly making breathing difficulty. The chapter on exercise delves into this in more detail.

Benefits of Proper Breathing

Here are some of the most important benefits of proper breathing.

1. Improved breathing allows for greater body efficiency, as there is an increase of oxygen in the bloodstream. This allows for improved brain and muscle function. For golfers, this could result in 10–15% improved yardage per shot and a decreased change of mishits.

1. Proper breathing allows the body to remove toxins and body wastes from the body. This allows for improved health and decreases the risk of injury.

2. Proper breathing allows for improved concentration and mental clarity. Golf requires extra clarity and concentration, without which one can more easily make a mistake or poor shot.

3. Proper breathing can be extremely important for controlling emotions. A terrible shot, a bad lie, or a difficult hole does not have to ruin an entire round. One can release the stress and move on to the next shot.

4. Proper breathing can increase energy, reduce stress, and decrease fatigue. With more oxygen, the cells are more efficient allowing for the body to move more easily.

5. Proper breathing can help with insomnia. A bad night's sleep can be terrible for the next round of golf.

6. Tip: Practice taking 100 deep breaths daily. They don't have to be all at the same time but can be done throughout the day. You can do 5–15 at a red light during your commute.

Breathing Exercises

The exercises described here are an important part of improving your golf game. The first exercises can be done twice a day. You can also do them if you find yourself having upsetting thoughts. Start this exercise by lying down on your back.

1. Place one hand on your chest and the other on your belly. When taking a deep breath, the hand on the belly should rise higher than the hand on the chest.

1. Exhale completely through your mouth.

2. Slowly take a deep breath in through your nose. Count to a number up to seven.

3. Exhale slowly through your mouth for a count up to eight. As the air is released, gently contract your abdominal muscles to completely remove the remaining air from your lungs.

4. Repeat this cycle for a total of five breath cycles.

The second exercise is similar to the first. This exercise takes a bit longer, and you hold your breath for four to seven counts between inhaling and exhaling. You can do this exercise anywhere, but a quiet place is preferable. Many of our patients do this exercise in their cars while stuck in traffic.

1. Exhale completely through your nose.

1. Slowly inhale through your nose, counting to a number up to seven.

2. Hold your breath for up to seven counts.

3. Exhale slowly through your nose for a count up to eight.

4. You will probably want to inhale air immediately. Try to inhale through your nose slowly and in a steady fashion.

5. Repeat up to ten times.

These exercises form the basis for the relaxation exercises in the next chapter.

Chapter Summary

- Breathing is an important part of life. High levels of oxygen allows for improved muscle function and performance.

- Breathing exercises can help calm oneself after a difficult hole or shot.

- Increased capacity means improved recovery times. This is important with breathing, as one can better recover one's heart rate and respiration rate, thereby not missing a critical shot.

Chapter 3

Sleep Your Way to a Better Golf Game

Breathing by itself doesn't help you hit better golf shots; you have to translate that breath into a physical change. A relaxation response needs to occur. Most people think of relaxation as lying on a couch watching football. In fact, if one is rooting for a particular team while watching, it will have the exact opposite effect. Relaxation changes how our bodies respond to stress. With that change, we have less tightness in our body, reduced cortisol, increased focus, and greater mental clarity. In this chapter we will discuss what relaxation means physiologically and how sleep is an important part of relaxation. An explanation of how the nervous system works in relation to stress and how you can affect it to gain benefits for your golf game. To start, let's discuss one of the most important relaxation techniques called sleep.

Sleep: Why it Matters

Sleep is a critical factor to performance, and not just the night prior to an event. Most Americans are sleep deprived. Recent studies say that over one-third of Americans do not get enough sleep. What happens when we don't get enough sleep? Generally, we feel fatigued, have trouble concentrating, and sometimes our mood drops.

Sleep can definitely affect athletic performance too, and in professional athletes a lack of sleep correlates to a player's inability to remain with the same team. Sleep deprivation increases injury risk, raises cortisol levels leading to weight gain, increases the risk of depression, decreases concentration, increases the risk of heart attacks, and other ill effects. Many memory problems in older adults are due to problems with sleep.

What is enough sleep? At least 8 hours is required and ideally 2 of those hours are before midnight. In several studies, people who slept from 10:00 pm to 6:00 am performed better than those who slept from midnight to 8:00 and had fewer health problems. For my patients who are executives, they like the before midnight rule. In general, executives are early risers so going to bed early allows them to not only rise early but also be at top form. For golfers, a bad night's sleep can cost as many as 3–5 strokes per round.

Of course, getting good sleep is easier said than done. Many people want to sleep more and do many things well to sleep better but just do not. There are a variety of factors for sleep disturbances. There are several issues that can arise from trouble falling asleep to waking early and everything in between, so let's discuss all of them. To understand why one may be having trouble with sleep, we will first need a discussion about cortisol.

Cortisol, Stress, and You

Cortisol is a hormone made by the adrenal glands that is responsible for helping one deal with stress. It cycles throughout the day, and in healthy people it should be highest in the morning and begin to decrease throughout the day. People under high stress (which can include athletes and executives) tend to have higher cortisol than others. Cortisol is also responsible for moving sugar out of storage and into the bloodstream.

Cortisol, in short bursts, helps us deal with a problem or situation through improved memory, increased attention, decreased pain sensitivity, and a quick burst of energy. When used in small amounts it can be very helpful. If cortisol is released continuously, then the relaxation response can decrease resulting in chronic stress. This can then lead to chronic disease that may include heart disease, decreased sleep, thyroid issues, blood sugar imbalances, weight gain, high blood pressure, decreased immunity, and more abdominal fat at the expense of muscle. (This is part of the benefit for meditation and neurofeedback that increases the relaxation response.)

Cortisol can be raised due to a variety of factors including, a lack of sleep, not eating properly or at the proper time, not drinking enough water, working out too much or too hard, working out late at night, and constant worry. Heavy anaerobic exercise, whereby the maximum heart rate gets too high can also lead to cortisol problems. This is less of an issue with golfers, but it can lead to a wired and tired state in someone who works out too heavily.

Sleep Disturbances

Persistently high levels of cortisol can lead to the first issue that can arise with sleep, the problem of falling asleep. Some people have difficulty only under certain circumstances, such as when they are too hot or they are nervous before a big event/match. This is actually fairly typical.

Generally, one should fall asleep in about 15 minutes from lying down. If you aren't falling asleep within 15 minutes, there is likely an imbalance in the body. When cortisol is too high late in the day, you will have difficulty falling asleep. An occasional issue is generally not a problem with cortisol. But if you find that you consistently take 30–60 minutes (or more) to fall asleep, you likely have a cortisol problem.

Learning to calm yourself to sleep better can be a chore. Medical attention can help, but taking a drug isn't a permanent solution. For one thing, it doesn't deal with the underlying issue. Solving the problem (as opposed to masking it) is an important step to total health. The other issue with many pharmacological sleep aids is that they just don't work. While most people do sleep, the quality of sleep tends to be poorer. Many people report feeling drugged the next day. Later in the book, we discuss ways to approach treatment of this issue, but it generally requires balancing cortisol.

Another common issue is waking often during the night. There are several variations of this problem, including waking and not going back to sleep, waking a lot to go

to the bathroom, waking due to leg cramping or jerking, waking too early, waking yourself up due to snoring (or someone waking you because you are snoring), waking in pain, and waking the same time every night. Each of these problems originates for different reasons.

Waking to go to the bathroom every night may be normal. As we get older, we may have an inability to hold our urine as long. For men, prostates enlarge and that can put pressure on the bladder giving one the feeling to urinate. In this situation, it is more likely that one will go to the bathroom several times a night. It is not normal however to do this constantly. Once a night is very different than waking even three times a night. When that occurs, there is probably an issue with your ability to concentrate urine, a function that resides in the adrenal gland through aldosterone.

Aldosterone is a hormone produced by the adrenal glands that helps the body retain sodium and potassium. Aldosterone should be higher during the night, but when our adrenals become imbalanced, aldosterone drops, which causes us to urinate more often than we should. With some people who have adrenal issues, aldosterone can be affected causing frequent nighttime urination. This is typically more than two or three times a night, but a mild version of this may cause someone to feel as if they need to urinate when lying down, even if they just relieved themselves.

Another common problem with urination occurs due to lactic acid. Lactic acid build up is common in athletes who do anaerobic exercise. Muscles produce lactic acid when working, and under conditions where there is enough oxygen, it is broken down further. When there is not enough oxygen (such as in sprinting), it builds up. Frequent urination occurs because lactic acid build-up irritates the

bladder wall. In this situation, we may wake or get up often to urinate but only have a small amount of urine come out. If you work out late at night, this could be the issue.

Lactic acid problems may occur due to more serious health concerns. Heart disease, kidney failure, or liver disease all can lead to high levels of lactic acid. Normally, the liver breaks down excess lactic acid, and if it is not doing its job properly, it will go the kidneys. Lactic acid may also build up from the heart not getting enough oxygen. If you are getting up a lot to urinate with small amounts of urine and haven't been exercising strenuously, it is best to see your doctor.

Sleep and Repairs

Why do we sleep at all? There are many theories to that, but one definitive reason is the repair of the body. This process can be disrupted, leading to sleep disturbances. During the night our body should increase anabolic activity to rebuild tissue and heal organs. In this state, the body is doing repairs and building things back up. It needs an appropriate amount of energy in the form of glycogen that is stored in the liver to do this work. The liver also stores appropriate amino acids that are used as building blocks to these repairs. Amino acids are the individual components of proteins.

When stores are not replenished, waking can occur in the middle of the night due to cortisol spikes. The body is looking for these stores to facilitate repairs. When we do not eat properly through the day or eat too close to our bedtime, we may not have adequate amounts of glycogen and amino acid stores to properly perform anabolic functions. The body may go into catabolism, the process

that breaks things down in the body, to give energy to the body. This generates hunger through higher levels of cortisol and epinephrine (adrenaline) and you will wake up at 4:00 a.m. ready to eat everything in the kitchen.

Cortisol Spikes at Night

Awakening at night because of cortisol (or more likely, adrenaline) can happen for reasons other than hunger. Bad dreams, high levels of stress, and anticipation of an event the next day can all create this response. The stress of long hours on the job can manifest as waking in the middle of the night. A fight with a co-worker or difficulty with a project can create unconscious problems. This is a different situation than the difficulty falling asleep, for in that situation the person's cortisol levels were high prior to going to bed whereas in this situation they likely fell asleep with no problem. The spike in cortisol in the middle of the night is an important clue that there is something else happening in your body. Meditation can be helpful for understanding anything that may be unresolved. More will be discussed in the chapter on meditation.

Pain can be another cause of cortisol spiking. Some people are able to control the response to pain such that falling asleep is not an issue. I have had patients where insomnia was the only sign of injury. During sleep, conscious suppression of pain is not possible and lying in a particular position may exacerbate the pain. Sleep is required to heal injuries, but if you are being awoken due to the pain, the depth of sleep is compromised such that you are unable to gain healing benefits. Treatment is necessary at this point and the chapter on treatments goes into great detail about this. Neurofeedback, cold laser, and manipulative-type adjustments to the body can greatly assist the healing.

Sleep and Diet

As discussed briefly in the chapter on diet, sleep can be affected by what we eat and drink. How often have you woke in the middle of the night after drinking red wine? Some foods can either spike cortisol in the middle of the night or there may be inflammatory properties to particular foods that cause waking. For some people, high amounts of sugar prior to bed can cause this spike due to the dreaded sugar crash. Alcohol can also create this problem. This is so prevalent that some doctors have Type 2 diabetics drink beer in the evening to bring blood sugar back down to a normal level by the morning. In a non-diabetic patient, that same beer causes a person to awaken due to the low blood sugar.

Food sensitivities can have a similar effect as well. The chapter on diet discusses this some, but suffice to say that a food that is irritating to the body can create a stress response. Cortisol elevation is part of the response, and if this occurs during sleep, it will disturb that activity. Some of our patients find their sleep improves on a detoxification diet for this reason. With better sleep, they tend to have better weight loss, which is an added bonus. These sensitivities may be increasing risk of injury, create increased brain fog, and otherwise interfere with one's ability to score well on the golf course.

The Timing of Waking

When a patient comes to the clinic complaining of waking, I always ask them what time. I usually get a look that says, "who cares?" but it can be indicative of a completely different type of imbalance. In classical Chinese medicine (CCM), the meridian system explains how the timing of waking can be significant. Depending upon the time one awakens, a different reason is assigned to the waking.

CCM describes the body as having 5 elements that correspond to an organ system. Each system is paired, creating 10 systems that are broken down on a 24-hour clock into 2-hour intervals. (There is one other paired system making up the other 4 hours, but we will ignore this for now.)

Consistently waking at the same time often corresponds to a problem existing in that system. Given that sleep occurs at night, the systems that can be disrupted are gall bladder, liver, lung, and large intestine.

In CCM parlance, 11:00 p.m to 1:00 a.m. is "gall bladder time." Waking in this time frame, or an inability to fall asleep at this time, may be reflected in problems with the gall bladder's function. For some people it may be related to the physical gall bladder in terms of their ability to process caffeine and fats. These people will often complain of right shoulder pain and an inability to eat fatty foods. They may have problems making decisions as well. For a golfer this could be reflected in debating which club to use for every shot not on the green. If this is a problem, eating fast food or Chinese food will produce pain or discomfort. Even if you have had your gall bladder removed, you could still be having problems with that organ from a CCM perspective.

Between 1:00 a.m. and 3:00 a.m. is "liver time." Waking consistently during this time period can have a variety of meanings. The liver is responsible for so many detoxification processes that awakening at this time could be related to the physical liver. Medications and alcohol can affect the liver and cause waking at this time. One pattern we have commonly seen is that the athlete who takes NSAIDs due to pain often wakes at this time. In this situation, the liver is overloaded. The liver also clears hormones and if it is not functioning properly, one may awaken at this time during high hormone times of one's cycle or with high levels of stress. The emotion associated with liver according to this philosophy is anger; unresolved anger can increase the likelihood of waking in this time frame. Some of my patients report having dreams about anger or being angry and waking between 1:00 a.m. and 3:00 a.m.

"Lung time" is between 3:00 a.m. and 5:00 a.m., and waking can occur due to issues with breathing and sinus issues. Patients with allergies or other sinus issues often awaken during this time period. Snoring can also be an issue during this time period, discussed below. In CCM, lung is paired with grief and sadness. Many of our patients who have had a recent loss will wake during this time. In some cases, the patients would wake crying at this time. This time period could also have something to do with cortisol, as it starts to rise around 4:00 a.m.

Finally, 5:00 a.m. to 7:00 a.m. is "large intestine time." Some people complain they wake at 5:00 or 6:00 and can't get back to sleep. Or they may wake and need to defecate. In many cases, food sensitivities or bad gut bacteria (a condition called dysbiosis) may be culprits. Most Americans, particularly athletes, eat too many refined carbohydrates leading to a variety of gut problems. Waking during this time may be the body's way of communicating this information.

Twitching and Cramping During Sleep

Twitching or jerking in one's sleep is also a somewhat common issue. Some athletes report their legs or arms jerking around when falling asleep. I have seen couples where one member of the pair complains that the other jars them out of bed. This could be a sign of over-training. Abrupt twitching generally is related to high levels of stress in the body. It is a clear sign that more rest and aerobic exercise is needed rather than anaerobic exercise. For some people, a lack of breathing is the problem and the chapter on breathing discusses this in great depth.

Similar to twitching some people wake with cramps. In most cases this occurs in the calves and is called a charley horse (in the U.S.). Generally the body isn't utilizing calcium, magnesium, and/or potassium properly. Potassium issues are rare in this situation as most will present with heart ailments. Calcium is associated with athleticism as it aids muscle contraction and when low can lead to muscle cramping. Magnesium though is the primary culprit in these situations, as we generally do not get enough in our diets. Foods that are high in magnesium such as chocolate or coffee are also high in biochemicals that leach the body of the same mineral. For sleep and cramping though, magnesium can be effective for both problems. When having trouble falling to sleep proper magnesium supplementation can aid the body in relaxing and calming it to better sleep. It appears to help cramping and certain formulations will help almost immediately.

As one starts a new exercise regime, one may have issues with achy joints. Waking with achy joints is not uncommon in this situation. Persistence of the problem though could be indicative of mineral deficiencies including calcium and magnesium. Some people also wake with headaches. In severe cases, this occurs in the middle of the night and can be a problem with dehydration. If water is not the issue, blood sugar may be too low. Some people don't get enough protein during the day causing a big drop at night. If the problem isn't solved with simple interventions, a visit to your healthcare provider would be in order.

Snoring

Snoring is another common complaint and can be a sign of other health issues resulting in health problems and poor sleep. Many problems that result in snoring include inflammation, hormone imbalances, digestive irritation, and allergies. For some people, losing weight will solve the problem of snoring. Others will require assistance in the form of a mouth guard to allow for the tongue to have increased space in the mouth or a CPAP machine. In other cases, snoring is just a sign of over-training. If it persists after backing off it is time to see a doctor for further workup.

As stated at the beginning of the chapter, improved sleep leads to an improved game. Don't allow your game and health to suffer when the issue can easily be corrected.

Waking at the Proper Time

No discussion about sleep would be complete without some words about waking at the proper time. With a good night of sleep one should awaken feeling refreshed and ready to start the day. A lack of this feeling could be due to a lot of different issues. Over training is a common cause of waking tired. People who are going too hard will not receive enough recovery in the night to feel fully rested. The body may not have completed all of the healing mechanisms and be attempting to tell one that it is important to take it easy that day so it can finish the job. In other cases, there is a high level of toxicity whereby the liver and kidneys have not completed all of the processes of detoxification. Molecules in interim states can lead to fatigue and weariness. In some cases, mental acuity may be hampered as well.

Along these lines, one may have food sensitivities contributing to fatigue and feelings of not being rested. Many of our patients find this situation disappears when doing a detox diet. Without the offending foods being consumed, the body isn't working hard to remove the toxins and other healing processes can occur. Foods that are toxic to a person can induce higher levels of cortisol or interfere with adrenal function in other ways. The adrenals are much like the battery in your car: if it's not working, you'll have trouble starting the car in the morning.

Consider the Environment when Sleeping

Getting proper sleep requires the proper environment. As stated at the beginning of the chapter, healthy sleep consists in getting an appropriate amount of sleep, sleeping some prior to midnight, and waking rested. But how does one prepare oneself to do this? We live in a fast-paced, intense environment with lots of conveniences for making our lives easier, but not necessarily for making them slower. There are many opportunities for distraction including cell phones, computers, television, and shopping malls. We can always find something to do. Electronic devices have a tendency to "wire us," which provides less than optimal conditions in our brains for sleeping. Allowing our brains to relax prior to bed is a great way to help with sleep. Generally, engaging our brains helps the most. One would think that doing something menial such as cleaning the house would be beneficial to shutting the brain down. Actually the opposite happens as it arouses the brain and makes falling asleep more difficult. Reading something mundane is excellent for this and probably explains why so many people fall asleep reading textbooks. In general, I recommend not having electronic devices (other than a cordless telephone) in your bedroom. Eliminate the television, computers, and so forth and see how your sleep can improve.

Another factor to assist in good sleep is a good mattress. While it may be obvious, having something that is comfortable and doesn't cause you to roll if anyone else is in the bed is an excellent choice. There are many models/types to choose from and this is not intended to be a review of such. Look for what is comfortable to all parts of your body while lying in different positions that you sleep. If it hurts in the store, it will certainly hurt at home.

Finally, keeping your room in darkness is very important to maintaining sleep hygiene. This can be challenging depending upon where you live. Summertime in the northern latitudes can create problems for one's sleep. Sunset at 10:00 or 11:00 p.m. combined with sunrises at 4:00 or 5:00

a.m. disrupts one's body clock. Blackout curtains and/ or eyeshades are excellent choices to assist this situation. These are recommended at all latitudes as ambient lights from city living can have the same effect as if one lived in northern Alaska in the summertime. Our bodies need darkness to turn on our healing mechanisms while we sleep, which can be disrupted by ambient light.

Just as living in higher latitudes in the summer can be disruptive, living at the same latitudes in the winter can be equally problematic. For many people awakening in the winter can be difficult as there is no light in the morning. In Portland, where I reside, the darkest days of winter can be miserable for patients as they arise early in the morning before the sun rises (which can't be seen anyway as there is a layer of rain clouds blanketing the city), and then the sun sets around 4:00 p.m. This doesn't provide for a lot of exposure to the sun, which is so important for our minds, bodies, and spirits. Aside from the obvious vitamin D deficiency, there are likely countless processes that require sunlight that we don't even know about. A full spectrum light is invaluable for getting through these really dark days. Twenty to thirty minutes in the morning can help the body activate processes. I have even recommended these types of lights for patients who live in Los Angeles and other places in lower latitudes.

Autonomic Nervous System

Hopefully you have a better understanding of the importance of sleep and how sleep can improve your golf game. Sleep improves brain function, reduces the risk of injuries (which prevent you from practicing), and allows for muscles to rest and repair. Having discussed sleep hygiene and issues with awakening, it is important to return to the general topic of relaxation. Relaxation is a process of letting go. This process changes our neurological response and affects our health in a variety of ways. If this process does not occur, long-term problems can result. To better explain this, a quick overview of the autonomic nervous system is important to create a frame of reference.

The autonomic nervous system (ANS) is responsible for activating many parts of our body below the level of consciousness. It affects heart rate, digestion, respiration, salivation, pupil dilation, urination, and sexual arousal. The ANS is basically divided into two main parts, the parasympathetic and sympathetic nervous system. The chart at the end of the chapter describes some of the basic functions attributed to each. One way to think about this is to imagine the accelerator and the brake on a car. The sympathetic nervous system is like the accelerator. It generally speeds things up in the body during a fight or flight response. Sympathetic dominance allows the body to prepare to hunt. The heart rate pumps faster and air passages are more open to better chase prey, pupils dilate for better vision, the liver pumps more glucose into the blood stream, the digestive system shuts down so that energy can be diverted out to the limbs and brain, the adrenal glands produce more adrenaline to continue the fight or flight response.

The parasympathetic nervous system does the opposite. It slows things down in the body. It prepares the body to be able to relax, repair and prepare for the next time the body needs to become active. It is preparing for the body to better assimilate the food that was just caught and eaten. It slows the heart rate down, produces more saliva, constricts the pupils, turns digestion on so that nutrients can be absorbed and waste eliminated. It is the preparatory phase for the body.

There are times when one of parasympathetic or sympathetic becomes overloaded and dominates the other. In parasympathetic dominance there isn't enough "oomph" to the person. Lethargy, a lack of motivation, and inability to engage in life dominate the person's life.

Most modern people have too much sympathetic activity. We are always in a hunting mode even when we are doing activities that are not governed by hunting. Our digestion is turned off even though we are eating big meals and not digesting those meals leading to indigestion. Our heart rate and blood pressure are higher. We are producing more adrenaline and cortisol (and gain weight as a consequence.) Over time this taxes the body creating many problems throughout. In other words, we are stressed. Research is showing that this high level of stress leads to many diseases of today such as heart disease and cancer. This high level of stress leads to increased inflammation. Reducing this imbalance is important for one's health.

Relaxation has the goal of increasing parasympathetic tone. We want to relax to allow our bodies to be able to turn down the processes that we are not using and turn on the processes that will help reduce the problems we are having. The big issue that we see has to do with digestion. People with sympathetic dominance tend to be gassy, prone to ulcers, and/or indigestion, eat fast and don't absorb nutrients very well. For most people the stress is in their heads.

Most of my physiology textbooks discuss the sympathetic nervous system by giving an example of escaping from a saber-toothed tiger. I was always amused by this example given that it had been 10,000 years or more since the last one of that species roamed the planet. But in some ways it is an excellent example. In modern society, the stresses of the day are less about survival and more in our perceptions. Our physiology doesn't distinguish between what is real and what isn't, as evidenced by how sweaty one's palms can get in the middle of a scary movie. We respond the same way regardless of the fact that the stress is imminent or something we are thinking about from the past.

More than any other athlete, golfers need a balance between the two parts of the autonomic nervous system. If you have too much parasympathetic tone, you will not have the stamina nor will there be enough engagement in the game to do well. Too much sympathetic tone and you will swing too hard, be too amped up, and be less likely to recover from bad shots.

As with driving however, balance between acceleration and braking is important. Both are required for optimal functioning. The yogis of the past understood how difficult it is to relax and therefore built it into their systems of health. Relaxation techniques vary depending upon what state one is in. For people who are stuck in a sympathetic mode, relaxation techniques that help quiet one down are most important. Turning things off, one's mind, phone, and television are all required for these people. Many executives are this type and find that going on vacation is the only thing that allows them to slow down. Interestingly, many management books suggest that to be more productive taking time off is key. Often these books cite CEOs who are able to delegate, work shorter hours, and leave work at the office as being the most productive and successful. This allows the highly driven person to not only slow down and recharge but to also gain perspective for their situation.

Being stuck in one ANS mode can limit choices. Sympathetic dominance makes everything an emergency; one cannot see the forest for the trees. Immediate action must be taken, as that is the realm of the sympathetic. In fight or flight mode, we don't always make the best decision. It is excellent for the hunt (or being hunted), but in relationships, business, and other life situations, the ability to step back and gain perspective is important. We may artificially limit choices because we see the situation as life or death. Slowing down allows for one to respond from a different place. For example, a parent may be playing with their five-year-old child and gets hit in the head by their child. The adult in sympathetic dominance may respond with aggressive action without realizing that they are being inappropriate. With balance, the same adult will realize that it was an accident or see that the child is just acting their age. The same situation leads to two different outcomes, but the appropriate response started by being relaxed and in balance.

For the golfer, the tension created by water is very familiar. A shot over water can cause the best golfer to tense up and not hit a good shot. In many ways, hitting over water is no different than hitting any other shot. We make it worse in our minds because there isn't room for error. But the same shot, same distance, and the same lie, without water doesn't bother us. Understanding the concepts of relaxation is extremely important for success in this situation.

Relaxations Exercises

Knowing something about the need to relax, what are some techniques to help one relax? There are many different exercises. Reading in bed is a perfectly good relaxation technique for some people. Relaxation is important to balance the autonomic nervous system, the parasympathetic, and sympathetic. Slowing down facilitates this process. Relaxation allows the body to adapt quickly to a situation.

Complete Body Relaxation

This technique can be used on the golf course if you become anxious. Several studies have shown this to be highly effective in helping people score better playing golf. Obviously you don't want to lie down on the golf course but the general concept can be done in a pinch. It is also an excellent way to prepare your body for sleeping just before bedtime.

1. Lie down on your bed or floor.

2. Using the breathing techniques from the previous chapter, take easy and deep breathes.

3. Tighten the muscles in your toes. Hold for a count of ten then release the tension. Notice how you feel.

4. Next tighten the muscles in your feet and hold for a count of ten. Release the tension.

5. Move up through each muscle group in your calves, your thighs, buttocks, back, abdomen, arms, legs, neck, and head.

6. Notice how you feel after each section and how the tension leaves your body.

Nervous System Table

Structure	Sympathetic Stimulation	Parasympathetic Stimulation
Iris (eye muscle)	Pupil dilation	Pupil constriction
Salivary Glands	Saliva production reduced	Saliva production increased
Oral/Nasal Mucosa	Mucus production reduced	Mucus production increased
Heart	Heart rate and force increased	Heart rate and force decreased
Lung	Bronchial muscle relaxed	Bronchial muscle contracted
Stomach	Peristalsis reduced	Gastric juice secreted; motility increased
Small Intestine	Motility reduced	Digestion increased
Large Intestine	Motility reduced	Secretions and motility increased
Liver	Increased conversion of glycogen to glucose	
Kidney	Decreased urine secretion	Increased urine secretion
Adrenal medulla	Norepinephrine and epinephrine secreted	
Bladder	Wall relaxed	Wall contracted
	Sphincter closed	Sphincter relaxed

Chapter Summary

- Sleep is extremely important to a good golf game, as it helps prevent injury, allows for muscle repair, and keeps brain function working optimally so that better decisions can be made on the course.

- There are many reasons as to why sleep can become disrupted, some having to do with cortisol levels in the body.

- Consider diet and over exertion as two possible problems related to sleep disturbances.

The body has two branches to the automatic processes, and relaxation is the process of balancing the sympathetic and parasympathetic nervous systems.

Chapter 4

Elevate Your Mind, Elevate Your Game

The famous golfer Bobby Jones once said, "Golf is game played on a five-inch course—the distance between your ears." What is the single most important part of playing golf? Golf at its core is a mental game. Learning to swing correctly is definitely a big part of the game. But being able to hit the ball well at the driving range and translate that into a good score on the course requires much more than a good swing.

Conditions on the course vary from game to game, which requires a different mindset for each shot. Focus and concentration are key to a good game, and one of the best ways to improve those is meditation. Players have all sorts of challenges on the course that they don't face on the driving range including first tee shot jitters, putting yips, and freezing during difficult shots. Meditation calms the mind down, which in turn allows the body to be calmer and improves your golf game. It allows you to better control these negative thoughts and play through them. Let's explore how this unfolds from the mental side and the physiologic side.

The Power of Positive Thinking

Most people when they play golf have what the Buddhists call, "monkey mind." Their minds are in chaos and always thinking. When addressing the ball, a golfer often thinks about their swing, what they want to do with their arms, think about the turn, or where they don't want to hit the ball. Their minds are anything but quiet. The average golfer thinks about what they don't want to do instead of what they do want to do. In general, we are more likely to manifest what we are thinking about, whether positive or negative.

Just for a second, I want you to remember the last time you were faced with a shot over water. Did you take out an old golf ball? Were you thinking, "I don't want to hit this into the water?" The subconscious ignores the negation in the sentence, interpreting, as "I want to hit this into the water." These types of thoughts and actions cause our bodies to tighten up and our muscles to work in a way that causes the action to come true. In this case, the thoughts, the actions, and the muscle tightening leads to the ball being shot into the water. Meditation allows one to learn to quickly reboot their brains and clear these negative thoughts. This allows you to approach each thought, each moment, with a clear mind.

Meditation is the ability to focus on one thing, the act of emptying one's mind. The focus can be on anything or nothing; your breath, an object, putting, a spiritual idea, a beautiful view. The intention of focus is less important than it being singular in purpose in the present moment.

For most of us, this is difficult, especially when we first start. Our mind is racing all over from one thought to the next. Our goal is to bring our focus back to the current moment. If you hit a bad shot or a good shot, it doesn't matter if you come back to the current moment. If you hit a great tee shot on a par 4, patting yourself on the back for that great shot won't help you hit the next shot near the pin. Meditation is about being in the now. Let go of the last shot and prepare for the current one.

Some Buddhist writers describe this process as similar to training a puppy to sit. When first starting, the puppy will not sit at all. Then it sits, but it gets up immediately. Eventually you tell the puppy to sit, and it sits and stays until you give it another command. You don't get frustrated or angry at the puppy; instead you patiently help it over and over again. Like the puppy, over time, you can train yourself to remove all extraneous thoughts in an instant and stay focused on one thing such as a putt, a tee shot, or difficult wedge pitch.

While meditation can be used in an instant, meditation primarily focuses on the process instead of the outcome. Jim Fannin is a coach that works with world-class athletes, including the 2011 PGA Player of the Year, Luke Donald. He trains people to have what he calls a "Champion Mindset." Mr. Fannin believes that the process is the core of the champion's mindset. Golf is a process. The paradox is that to score well in golf, one must embrace the process and let go of the result. While cliché, it is true that a good score happens one shot at a time. To play well, one must remember that not all of your shots will be perfect. Ben Hogan once said that he only hits four good shots in a round. Golf is the game of the imperfect, and if we try to be perfect, we will drive ourselves crazy. The goal of golf is to get par on each hole (or bogey or double bogey depending upon your handicap). For a scratch golfer on a par 3, it doesn't matter if the person hits a terrible tee shot and chips next to the hole for a 1-putt or a great tee-shot, and then hits 2 putts. While the process differs, there's still a 3 on the scorecard.

Meditation is about finding equilibrium. How many times have you started a round really well, then you start thinking about your score and it falls apart towards the end? Or conversely you start terribly, forget about the score, and then play great the rest of the way. This is due to our mind playing tricks on us. One cannot become too upset or too happy about any particular, shot, hole, or round. Meditation allows us to find that center. It is the act of letting go of thoughts. Through being able to maintain focus, there will be better clarity of the process and scoring will improve.

Physiologic Benefits of Meditation

While meditation is thought of as a mental activity, it has very specific beneficial effects on the body. The last chapter discussed relaxation and many people don't distinguish relaxation from meditation. It is important to understand the difference between the two, as there are separate physiologic responses to each. Whereas relaxation is a state whereby a person releases tension in their body and somewhat in the mind, meditation is a state of mental alertness. Relaxation balances the autonomic nervous system so that there is a balance between braking and acceleration. Meditation is about keeping the balance of awareness on a razor thin edge within the mind.

The benefits of meditation are enormous, as it has been shown to reduce stress, lower blood pressure, changes in hormone response, improved immune function, and a subjective correlation to improved mood and quality of life. Furthermore, meditation reduces injury and improves concentration. Meditation allows the mind to be more amenable to positive suggestions to play better. Both benefits will improve your game and allow you to play pain free.

Meditation has many other benefits to the mind and the body. First, meditation increases endurance in athletes. The mechanism of this isn't clear, but may have something to do with oxygen consumption. Meditation decreases oxygen consumption by 12–20% depending upon ethnicity and other factors. This reduces sensitivity to CO_2 and decreases respiration rate. In response, tissue metabolism also changes, causing a decline in arterial lactate levels. For an athlete this would likely decrease muscle cramping or pain associated with muscle usage. Also, increased lactate in the muscles and blood stream may be one cause of overuse injuries. These types of injuries are common amongst golfers. Strains, sprains, and pulled muscles are more likely to occur with elevated levels of lactate in the muscles. Meditation by itself won't prevent these injuries, but they could help reduce them when combined with the other principles mentioned in this book including proper diet and exercise.

Another benefit of meditation is the positive changes it creates in various hormone and neurotransmitter levels. Feel good neurotransmitters like serotonin and endorphins increase after meditation and stress hormones like epinephrine are generally reduced. These changes last for hours and can have longer-term effects with regular practice. Obviously, these types of changes can help one's game as feeling good, having less pain, and reduced stress all contribute to better performance.

The most striking benefits to meditation, however, appear to be in the brain. Electroencephalography (EEG) is a technique that allows researchers to look at how the brain's electrical activity is working. EEGs differ between people who do and do not meditate: the biggest change is that there is increased phase coherence meaning that the brain is working in a more synchronous pattern. This is generally associated with greater creativity and being in the "flow."

Being in the flow is difficult to describe. One way I have heard this explained is that a person will say they feel like things are clicking. The ability to solve problems, see solutions and make decisions all come easily.

In terms of golf, being in the flow is extremely important to the success of one's game. When one is in the flow of the game, one will hit shots that are not only well struck but also well placed. One doesn't have to think about the shot as much because the best approach can be seen clearly. Focus and concentration are enhanced. When not in the flow, one struggles with where to place the shot. One worries about the hazards in front of them. Meditation can allow a person to be more in tune with the game and the flow that makes them more successful.

How To Practice

How many times have you gone to the driving range, picked up a bucket of 100 balls and hit ball after ball mindlessly for 30 minutes? This is not a routine that will lead to better scoring. Good practice requires an approach that will simulate game time conditions as best as possible. Using the principle of meditation, we can use our practice time to improve muscle memory and create the game time mentality required to succeed on the course.

I like to break golf into two types of practice: mechanics and focus. The first type requires learning the correct swing motion and creating muscle memory for that type of movement. This requires taking a lot of swings, and analyzing each through watching the flight path of the ball. One takes a shot and through an understanding of the flight path of the ball, you can determine what needs to be corrected in the swing to fix the problem. If you don't know how to do this, you need lessons from a professional who can explain this to you so that practice becomes more effective. What practice shouldn't consist of is mindlessly hitting a shot to the right and immediately hitting another ball. It requires thought and awareness.

The only time that I will hit a large bucket of balls is when I'm working on a specific issue with my swing mechanics. Generally, I hit only 25–35 balls as I take lots of swings and if I miss a shot, I think about the trajectory and take the swing in slow motion 5–10 times until I feel that the movement is correct, and then I hit another shot. I take this approach to chipping practice as well. I go to the practice area and work on difficult lies. I only take 2–3 balls and take several practice swings. I then address the ball as if I'm on the course and going through my routine as if playing a round. If I don't hit a good shot, I work on a different one and come back to it. The only time I may hit many shots in a row is when I have a new club (usually a wedge) that I am trying to gauge distances to determine how to place the ball appropriately.

The second type of practice is one I recently discovered while on the course one day. I hit a terrible second shot on a par 4 after an amazing drive down the fairway. My immediate response was to reach into my bag and grab another ball. I didn't, but I realized that my thought process for practice was off. We tend to play the same way that we practice and the way I had been practicing had a do-over mentality to it. I started going to the range and instead of just hitting balls, I would imagine I was on the course and rotate through my clubs as if playing a hole. For example, I might imagine being on the first tee at Langdon Farms to start. From the white tee box, the yardage is 359 yards.

I usually start with my driver, so I hit that. I'd watch my shot and determine where it landed in terms of yardage left to the green and select another club to represent that shot. Then I would hit that club and continue this process until I was on the green. I sometimes would practice a chip as well if appropriate. What it doesn't really help with is playing conditions. Langdon Farms is a links-style course and has almost no even lies. Even when in the fairway the ground is not as level as a driving range mat. But this type of practice helps take away the mindless hitting of balls and requires one to have more thought about each shot. If you mishit the ball, you need to think about what it was that went wrong and how to correct it with a different club.

Once I changed my practice approach, my scoring improved. I was practicing more like how I needed to play and had more of a game mentality.

Types of Meditations

There are an infinite number of ways to meditate. It can be done while sitting, standing, walking, or lying down. Golf itself can be considered a meditation. One can use the quiet of one's mind to find something deeper within oneself. It can also be used to find stillness in other areas of one's life. Below we describe several meditation methods. The first is a foundation that can be used with the other methods. It allows one to calm and gain the benefits discussed above. The others are more specific to athletic performance. Visualizations can be used prior to a round or even during a round to increase focus and prepare for a shot.

Basic Meditation

The first type of meditation to discuss is Zen meditation. This is the best-known type of meditation in the West. Is it useful for golfers? Probably, as many pros including Tiger

Woods and Justin Rose use meditation as part of their routines. The technique is simple conceptually but difficult to master. It is best to start doing everyday for 5–10 minutes in the morning. This meditation can be done cross-legged if you are flexible enough. This is the foundation for all of the other meditations we will discuss.

1. Sit upright in a stool or hard-back chair with your feet on the ground and palms resting on your thighs.

2. Your eyes can be open or closed. Once comfortable, begin focusing on your breathing. Use one of the breathing exercises from the previous chapter or silently count from 1 to 10.

3. Keep your mind quiet for the duration of the exercise. As thoughts come to mind watch them as one may watch clouds go by.

4. Keep breathing gently without taking too deep of a breath.

It is best to start with only 5 minutes and then work your way up to 20 minutes.

Visualizations

Visualization is also important to golfers. As alluded to previously, when one visualizes their shot, one is more likely to make better shots. The simple act of visualizing a good shot improves your chances of making one. This exercise is specifically not golf related, but it can be helpful on the course.

1. Sit in a comfortable position with your feet firmly on the ground.

2. Close your eyes and imagine yourself somewhere peaceful. You want to create a place that is an inner oasis, a special place. It can be a temple, a beach, a spa, anything that is meaningful to you.

3. Breathe gently and easily. Add elements to your space that are appropriate. Visualize the details of the space that feel right.

4. If you want, you can add emotions to the visualization. You can feel safety, love, compassion, or anything else that feels right to you.

5. Continue for up to 25 minutes but no longer.

The previous exercise can be modified to go through a successful round as well. In this exercise, imagine yourself playing at a course you like to play or are about to play. Imagine hitting a perfect tee shot on the first hole. Go to the location of the ball and see yourself hitting a great second shot. Continue seeing yourself play the entire course exactly the way a professional might play it.

Chapter Summary

- Meditation provides for physiological changes in hormones, neurotransmitters, and muscle endurance that allows for improved play

- Through the power of mental alertness combined with stillness, our brain waves change, allowing for improved concentration and focus. This allows for improved play on the course.

- Meditation allows us to understand how our brains work and spot negative thoughts so they can be easily cleared and brought back into focus.

- While golf may be a form of meditation for some, other techniques may be used to bring ourselves into focus on the golf course.

Chapter 5

Strength, Flexibility, Balance: The Core of Improving Your Game

The final principle of yoga to be discussed is exercise. Golf is exercise, and as we see below it requires the use of most if not all of the muscles in the body to swing a club properly. What is it about yoga that is so helpful to golfers? Yoga provides the three basic physical requirements for a golfer: strength, flexibility, and balance. Through the practice of yoga, one can obtain all three. The increase in flexibility helps prevent injuries, as a lack of flexibility is the leading cause of injuries in golfers. The improvement of balance helps one's swing, as balance is integral to maintaining proper form, and the increased strength allows one to hit the ball further. To gain all of these benefits, a regular practice of yoga is necessary.

Yoga practice is a lot like playing golf: you have good and bad days. Some days you will feel extremely loose and supple. Getting into poses will be easy and graceful. Other days you will wonder why you are doing this at all and wish you didn't have to finish. It's all part of the process, and while it may or may not make you a better person, it will make you a healthier one.

As yoga is a process, it is important to do each step fully and not rush. Breathing evenly and deeply is important as you do each pose. Some poses seem to have a breathing pattern that is counter to typical patterns. That's okay. Be aware of that and keep breathing. Paying attention to your breath is important. It is the foundation for quieting your mind as well, the most important skill in anyone's golf game.

Yoga exercises are a form of meditation themselves, meaning it is bringing awareness to areas where there was none before. As you do each pose, you will most likely feel some pain. (See the note below about types of pain.) Breathe through that pain, and feel what parts of your body are tight. Feel any emotions you may be having, stay in that place, and don't judge. Often when we are doing poses our bodies lengthen and stretch causing our minds and feelings to do the same. I like to think of it as a biochemical release. (For more information about emotions being stored in the body, see Candace Pert's book, *Molecules of Emotion*) Emotions reside not in our brains, but rather throughout our bodies. As we stretch and lengthen, the stuck places open and release toxins, chemicals, and neurotransmitters. Some of those things are also emotions and as they are released we often experience them again. By paying attention (and drinking water) we can release them. This may be the most important part of improving your game. Through this practice, many people have learned about self-doubt and sabotaging beliefs that they were able to overcome. Yoga also gives you body awareness. This allows you to learn more about your positioning in space, which is critical in creating a good golf swing.

Muscles Used in Golf

I am often asked what muscles to work on to improve one's swing. The short answer is all of them. Golf is whole body exercise. Your ability to drive the ball long distances requires a tremendous amount of torque to your back and hips, so without proper preparation and stretching, driving can lead to long-term damage. Let's go through the muscle groups to better understand the mechanics. This has helped some of my patients understand their swings better. When working on the exercises it can be helpful to use visualization to increase flexibility and muscle mass.

Neck and Head: Proper alignment of one's neck is imperative to a good swing. If you are pulling your neck or picking your head up too quickly, you are likely to misdirect the ball. The muscles serve two purposes. The first is keeping the head still on the back swing but the muscles must be able to release and move the head forward on the follow through. This presents a one-way situation. In a right-handed golfer, the neck will only turn to the left potentially creating an imbalance between the two sides. The sternocleidomastoid (SCM) is the primary muscle used, but other muscles can be affected as well. Some patients complain of an inability to turn their neck to the right when backing up in a vehicle.

In Chapter 6, proper alignment will be discussed. With respect to the neck, the neck's role for humans is to maintain the eyes level to the ground. The neck may go out of alignment in response to misalignment in other parts of the body.

Shoulders: The shoulders are important in helping one rotate the torso and carry the club. These muscles along with the arms and chest help generate club speed during the swing. They also control the plane of the club. Shoulder muscles stabilize the arms and allow for the appropriate club path. Excessively tight shoulder, upper back, or chest muscles will prevent proper rotation of the back and cause an inability of arm extension throughout the swing.

Chest: The chest muscles help rotate the trunk, maintain club speed, and generate power. New golfers often find these the most tender after hitting some balls.

Upper Back: The upper back muscles allow for rotation of the trunk and lift of the golf club. They also carry the arms throughout the swing.

Lower Back: Also rotate the trunk and maintain position during the swing. This is a common area for injury due to the amount of torque placed on the area. Without flexibility in the lower back, the golfer will not be able to rotate properly during a swing.

Hips: The hips help rotate the trunk and generate power at ball impact. Hip tightness can affect the swing greatly because you cannot get a full rotation to hit the ball straight. Hip mobility is important as it affect the backswing and downswing. The hips are important for load and coil during the backswing and the release in the downswing. If the hips are limited in mobility, there will be too much lateral motion during the swing.

Upper legs: The upper legs generate power and maintain the swing position. These muscles help protect the lower back.

Abdominal Muscles: These balance your body and protect the lower back muscles. Strengthening your abdominal muscles allows you to generate more power through the rotation of the swing.

Lower legs: Calf muscles are excellent for providing balance and maintaining proper foot position. They assist with the backswing and follow-through. Other muscles in the lower legs help with toe positioning, which contributes to proper balance.

Upper Arms: These muscles help control the swing and maintain proper club position. Interestingly, the arms don't contribute much to the power of a golf swing. The power is generated from most of the other parts of the body.

Lower Arms: The muscles of the wrists and hands assist with gripping the club and maintaining proper position. The wrists are incredibly important for golfers. The right flexors and left extensors are the primary muscles used in the swing. Exercises are needed to balance the wrists after learning to swing a golf club. Stretches are important as well. Swing speed is generated as a result of the lower arms as well.

Types of Pain

When showing a patient these exercises one time, she commented how much it hurt. "This is really difficult," she said. "I am not comfortable at all!" She understood that while there was discomfort the pain wasn't unnatural.

Pain comes in many forms, from the physical to the emotional. For most people, physical pain is easy to recognize. You feel it in your body at a specific location. The intensity can vary from a mild discomfort to a searing, burning experience that makes you believe you are about to die. A well-done yoga pose in a healthy person can generate pain that is normal. When we stretch, creating greater flexibility and strength, we generally feel it. That type of pain typically burns in a specific location. For example, if you are doing bicep curls correctly, that muscle will become tight and engaged. If there is a lot of weight that you are lifting relative to your strength, it may burn as well. What it shouldn't feel like is radiating pain up your neck or down to your hand. You may feel the bicepital tendon at the shoulder but it won't click or burn. The tendon that attaches to the lower arm shouldn't click, burn, or feel a tearing sensation.

Preliminary Work

Prior to starting, one should determine if this would even be safe for a person to do. Here's a simple test. Can you do a Downward Facing Dog (Pose 4) without pain? I don't mean the stretch type of pain. If you can't, you need to do one or two weeks of warm-up exercises. You are in need of some serious stretching and the first week will be too hard for you. If after two weeks you don't feel very limber, it may be time for professional help. A yoga class or a visit to a healthcare professional may be in order to help. Otherwise, you could risk injury.

Another test is to determine if your hips are stable. Hip problems can lead to pain in other parts of the body due to the nature of the joint. The hip and sacrum pivots in such a way that one leg can appear to be longer than the other, causing rotation somewhere else in the spine. A simple test is to perform chair pose with your heels 2–4 inches off the ground. If you cannot keep your back straight in this position, the hip joint isn't stable and these exercises are definitely needed prior to starting the other routines. These exercises are also just helpful for strengthening the legs and pelvis, so they are recommended for anyone.

Hip Stabilization Exercises

These exercises are done in sequence one after the other. Do all the exercises on one side and then repeat on the other side. Between each exercise do not allow your raised foot to rest. Start with 5 repetitions of each sequence and work your way up to 20 per exercise per side. You want to do the same number on each side. These exercises will benefit most golfers. They stabilize the core and allow for greater balance. If you are balanced when golfing, even if you don't hit the ball flush, you are much more likely to hit a shot that carries well and is straight. Hip stabilization exercises helps with balance, as does yoga in general.

To start these exercises do the following:

- Lay on your side with your hip on the floor.

- Place your lower arm under your head propping it up and your upper arm on the floor to stabilize yourself.

- Start with your upper foot about 3–4 inches raised above your lower foot. This is neutral position.

- All the movements should originate from your upper hip.

- Maintain stability of your leg as it shouldn't move at all.

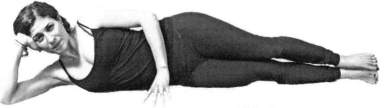

Side-lying Tiger Start

Side-lying Tiger

1. While keeping your leg parallel to the floor, slowly bend your leg until your upper leg is at a 90-degree angle in front of your hips and your lower leg is bent to a 90-degree angle at the knee. Bend the knee using the muscles from your hip.

2. Slowly straighten your leg while bringing your leg back behind your resting leg. Make sure you do not move your hips back and forth while doing this motion. There will be some movement based on the leg movement but use your leg only to do this exercise.

3. With each motion, ensure that your upper foot passes over your lower foot. In other words, your leg should be straight as it goes through the neutral position in both directions.

4. Continue until you reach your repetition limit.

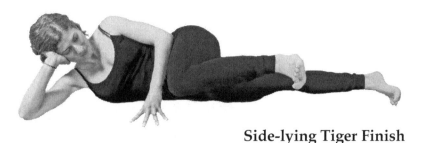

Side-lying Tiger Finish

Short Leg-Lift

1. Using the base of your leg, slowly lift your leg up about 4–6 inches higher than your starting position.

2. Slowly return your leg to the neutral position.

3. Continue until you reach your repetition limit.

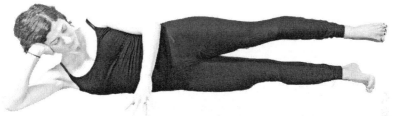

Low Leg Lift

Side-lying Tiger with Extension

1. While keeping your leg at the same level, bend your leg until your knee is at a 90-degree angle in front of your hips.

2. Once you reach the 90-degree position, extend your leg straight from that position.

3. Slowly straighten your leg while bringing your leg back behind your resting leg. Make sure you do not move your hips during this motion.

4. With each motion ensure that your upper foot passes over your lower foot. In other words, your leg should be straight as it goes through the neutral position in both directions.

5. Continue until you reach your repetition limit.

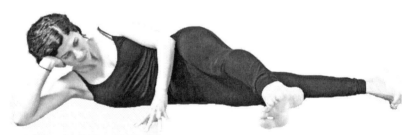

Side-lying Extension

High Leg-lift

1. From the base of your leg, lift your leg up about 10–12 inches higher than your starting position.

2. Slowly return your leg to neutral position.

3. Continue until you reach your repetition limit.

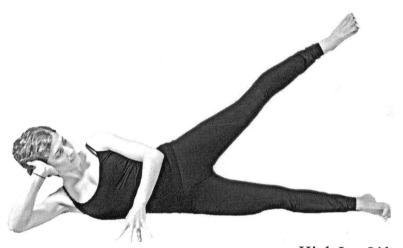

High Leg Lift

Side Lying Circle Rotations

1. Keeping your leg about 4–6 inches above your starting position.

2. From the hip joint, slowly rotate your leg in clockwise direction.

3. Continue until you reach your repetition limit and then continue going in a counter-clockwise direction.

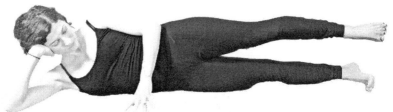

Side-lying Circle Rotations

The Exercise Routines

The program is designed to be a three-week program to get you started towards a healthier you. Why three weeks? It takes on average 21 days to start a new habit. Your challenge is to follow this regime for 21 straight days with no days off. If you have to take a day off, you need to start over again. For most people this won't be a problem. It's a simple matter of finding 15–30 minutes every day to stretch, relax, and meditate. After three weeks, taking a day or two off won't be a problem. You will have created the habit whereby you will be able to take one or two days off and go back to it. Often, people who do this feel something is off on their days that they don't do yoga. They just don't feel like themselves.

Where appropriate, we will discuss which poses can be lengthened for more of a stretch or more strength building. You will feel tightness in different parts of you body. If you haven't stretched your muscles in a long time, this will be uncomfortable. A little pain or even a lot of localized pain may be a good sign. That means that you are gaining a benefit. It is probably the pain that had you stopped stretching at some point in the first place. Working through this tightness is an important first step. For some people, working only on the preliminary poses is necessary for several weeks just to be loose enough to perform other exercises. This is not a problem. Go at the best pace for you to gain benefit while not creating harm to your body.

Below are a series of exercise routines that can be done in order to begin your yoga exercise experience. For each pose, we have an explanation of the pose and why it helps, the instructions for doing the pose, details about the position if needed, cautions about the pose, and the muscles that are generally worked. Sometimes people are very tight so the muscles worked may vary. Over time you should start feeling the pose in the muscles indicated. If you are not feeling the pose in those locations, then you may be doing the pose wrong or if you are feeling pain in other areas, there may be something else wrong and it is an indication to visit your healthcare provider.

Mixed Sequence: Sitting and Standing

Week one starts with poses that are designed to get the blood flowing and loosen the body. It is important to learn these well, as they will become the foundation for your practice in the future. Most of our patients benefit from this, as they are able to increase flexibility and strength at the same time. When starting out, it is generally best to go slow, and if your body is tight, gently work into the tightness. Do several sun salutations in a row lengthening the time between positions each time and going deeper into the stretch. This allows the body to warm up and stretching generally works better when the body is warm. Studies have found that if you stretch too much when the body is cold, you are at greater risk for injury.

Pose 1: Cat-Cow

Cat-Cow (also called Cat-Dog) is an excellent pose to begin to open and loosen your body. Some people go back and forth between the two slowly to get the blood flowing. Generally, this helps the lower back and shoulders. Most people hold their lower back sticking it out too much and their upper back goes back too much. Cat-Cow allows for a correction of both of these issues and introducing more extension (moving forward) in the upper back and more flexion (moving backwards) in the lower back. (See diagram). By doing this several times, you loosen the back allowing for more blood flow and start to warm the muscles that you use for swinging a club. This pose stimulates your kidneys and adrenals.

Instructions:

1. Come down unto hands and knees as if you are going to crawl.

2. While inhaling, tilt your sit bones up towards the sky. Draw your shoulder blades down your back and lift your gaze.

3. Exhale and round your spine towards the ceiling while lifting your navel (belly-button) towards your spine.

4. Do this 3–5 times.

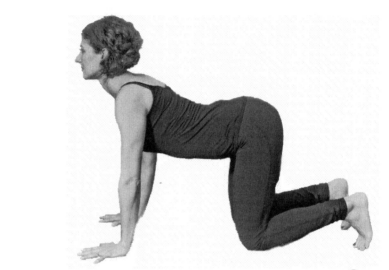

Cow

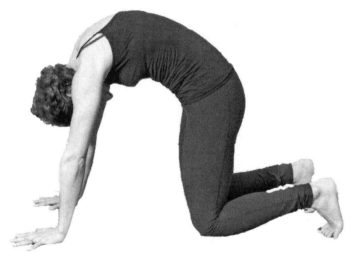

Cat

Position:

- Keep your hands under your shoulders and parallel to each other.

- Your knees should be shoulder width apart with your thighs perpendicular to the floor.

- While rounding your back go slowly and notice the tight areas. Those are the ones that you want to lengthen so that they get a complete stretch.

- Most golfers will feel cat in their lumbar region as they round the spine. By trying to lengthen that region a greater stretch will occur. Go easy though because if you stretch too much, too fast, you can hurt your back.

- You can also take several breaths in each position while lengthening your body. This deepens the stretch.

Cautions:

If your lower back is hurting intensely or you have pain, numbness, or tingling going down your leg, please visit your doctor immediately. While there may be tightness in the back, particularly in the lumbar region, that pain should be mild and under no circumstances should it radiate to another location below the back.

Recent or chronic injury to knees, shoulders or neck could make this pose difficult. Please consult with your clinician if this is the case.

Pose 2: Thread the Needle

This is a wonderful pose for opening your arms, shoulders, and releasing tension in your neck. This works the rotator cuff and neck muscles allowing for a gentle stretch of those muscles. Stretching these areas are very important before and after a round of golf.

Instructions:

1. From the above starting position, slide your left arm under your right, creating a bridge with your right arm.

2. Bring your right arm forward and form a 90-degree angle at the elbow.

3. Continue to slide your left arm under until you are resting both your left ear and your left shoulder on the mat.

4. Find the position where you feel the deepest stretch.

5. Hold the pose for 3–6 breaths and then do the other side.

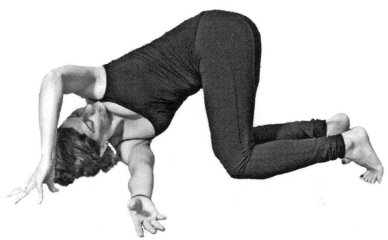

Thread the Needle

Position:

- Keep your shoulder and ear to the ground.

- Keep the non-threaded arm at a 90-degree hinge at the elbow. That arm will appear to be in front of you.

- Breathe gently as you do this.

Modifications:

Place a folded blanket under the knees to protect them from stress and pressure. Cross the upper hand over the back and hold onto the inside of the opposite thigh. This can generate more stretch.

Contraindications:

Recent or chronic injury to the knees, shoulders, or neck can be exacerbated by this pose.

Pose 3: Child's Pose

This pose is very good at any time. It gently stretches the lower back and tones the abdominal organs to stimulate digestion and elimination. It is a resting pose, which means that it can be used at any time. Some people use this to rest after a difficult series. It can also be used if your back is tightening a little. For a golfer, this pose stretches out the very lower back near the sacrum. This area can tighten up after a round. I like using this pose after a round to help release any tension there post workout.

Instructions:

1. From the Cat-Cow starting position, exhale and lower your hips towards your heels, insuring that your feet are flat on the floor.

2. Spread your knees apart slightly.

3. Extend your hands over your head while you bring your head down to the floor.

4. Hold the pose for 3–6 breaths.

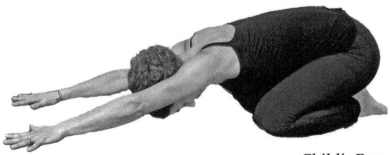

Child's Pose

Position:

- You should feel this in your lower back and your hips.

- Keep breathing into your belly as much as possible. This opens up the back and the sides.

- If your feet cramp, you can curl them such that the toes are under the floor.

- Keep your knees apart and your toes touching as if you are creating a V-shape with your legs.

Cautions:

If your lower back is hurting intensely or you have pain, numbness, or tingling going down your leg, please visit your doctor immediately. While there may be tightness in the back particularly in the lumbar region, that pain should be mild and under no circumstances should it radiate to another location below the back.

Contraindications:

Recent or chronic injury to knees, shoulders or neck could make this pose difficult. Please consult with your clinician if this is the case.

Pose 4: Downward Facing Dog

This pose calms your nervous system while engaging overall strength, flexibility, and decompressing your spine. It tones your arms and legs while stretching your hamstrings, calves and opening the arches of your feet. The first Downward Facing Dog you do in your practice is a good time to check in with how you are feeling that day. In my experience, I go much deeper after I have had time to move my body. Check in with how you are feeling and allow your body to lengthen if it feels right. You can always do the variation form so as not to pull muscles the first time through. Golfers can use this to stretch out one's back before or after a round of golf.

Instructions:

1. From Child's pose, place your hands to the floor about shoulder width apart.

2. Start curling your toes back under your feet and press into the floor.

3. As you press with your toes, press with your hands and start walking your feet toward the back of the mat. Use your hips to lift your body. Keep your knees well bent.

4. Tilt your sit bones up to lengthen your spine.

5. Press down further attempting to place your heels to mat as well, although most people cannot do this.

6. Breathe deeply and freely.

7. Hold the pose for 3–6 breaths.

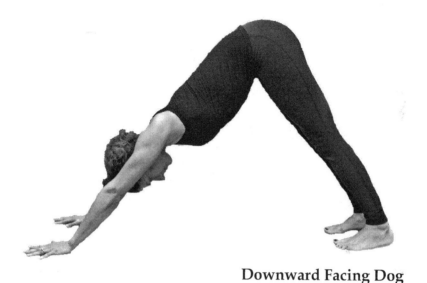

Downward Facing Dog

Position:

- Palms should be flat on the floor and fingers spread apart.

- Feel you thighs move back engaging your quadriceps.

- Pull your navel towards your spine.

- Tilt your tailbone up.

- Drop your shoulder blades down your back and bring your elbows in.

- Bring your ears in line with your upper arms. This protects your neck while elongating the spine.

- Your feet should be hip width apart.

Cautions:

If your lower back is hurting intensely or you have pain, numbness, or tingling going down your leg please, visit your doctor immediately. While there may be tightness in the back, particularly in the lumbar region, that pain should be mild and under no circumstances should it radiate to another location below the back.

Contraindications:

Very tight hamstrings can lead to a pulled hamstring. Go very gently if you have tight hamstrings and allow your body to warm up prior to going deeper into this exercise.

Wrists can also be strained with this pose, so if they are troubling you, press down through the knuckles of your index fingers. Use your whole body to bring the force out of your wrists. Move your thighbones back and engage them along with your core muscles.

Pose 5: Standing Forward Bend

This pose helps calm the brain and relieve stress. It stretches the hamstrings, calves, and hips. It also strengthens the thighs and knees. It can improve digestion. Mostly though this benefits the lower back. You can use the gluteals to lengthen the other muscles in the area that help support the lower back. It also helps release the piriformis muscle that when tight can create lower back issues. With release of these muscles, the follow through on the swing should be easier and more fluid.

Instructions:

1. From Child's pose, place your hands to the floor about shoulder width apart.

2. Start curling your toes back under your feet and press into the floor.

3. As you press with your toes, press with your hands and start walking your feet toward the back of the mat.

4. Tilt your sit bones up to length your spine.

5. Press down further attempting to place your heels to mat as well although most people cannot do this.

6. Breathe deeply and freely.

7. Hold the pose for 3–6 breaths.

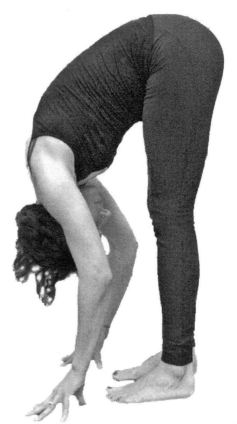

Standing Forward Bend

Position:

- Palms should be flat on the floor and fingers spread apart.

- Feel you thighs move back engaging your quadriceps.

- Pull your navel towards your spine.

- Tilt your tailbone up.

- Slightly rotate your thighbones outward. (Move the front of your thigh away from your body.) This creates more strengthening of the pelvic floor.

- Drop your shoulder blades down your back and bring your elbows in.

Cautions:

If your lower back is hurting intensely or you have pain, numbness, or tingling going down your leg, please visit your doctor immediately. While there may be tightness in the back, particularly in the lumbar region, that pain should be mild and under no circumstances should it radiate to another location below the back.

Contraindications:

Very tight hamstrings can lead to a pulled hamstring. Go very gently if you have tight hamstrings and allow your body to warm up prior to going deeper into this exercise.

Wrists can also be strained with this pose so if they are troubling you, can pressing down through the knuckles of your index fingers. Use your whole body to bring the force out of your wrists. If you move your thighbones back and engage them along with your core muscles, you will be able to remove some of the force from your wrists.

Pose 6: Halfway Lift

The halfway lift stretches the hamstrings, lower back, and tones the abdominal obliques. This pose is extremely important for golfers as the abdominal obliques are used a lot in a swing. Having strong stomach muscles helps prevent injury to the back. Finally, this pose helps lengthen the back throughout the spine.

Instructions:

1. From Standing Forward Bend, keep your feet together and place your fingertips on the floor.

2. Start curling your toes back under your feet and press into the floor.

3. As you press with your toes, press with your hands and start walking your feet toward the back of the mat.

4. Tilt your sit bones up to length your spine.

5. Press down further attempting to place your heels to mat as well although most people cannot do this.

6. Breathe deeply and freely.

7. Hold the pose for 3–6 breaths.

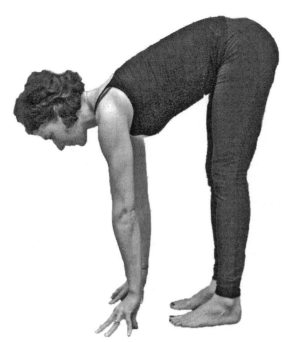

Halfway Lift

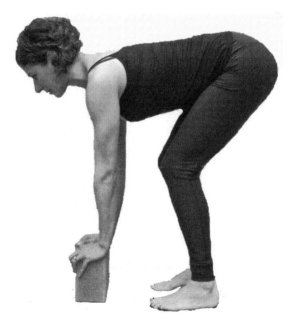

Halfway Lift Block

Position:

- Palms should be flat on the floor and fingers spread apart.

- Feel you thighs move back engaging your quadriceps.

- Pull your navel towards your spine.

- Tilt your tailbone up.

- Drop your shoulder blades down your back and bring your elbows in.

- Extend and lengthen your spine and bring your neck into alignment.

Cautions:

Very tight hamstrings can lead to a pulled hamstring. Go very gently if you have tight hamstrings and allow your body to warm up prior to going deeper into this exercise. Knees can be bent further to ensure a flat back.

Be careful if you've had a recent back injury because this can put a lot of pressure onto your lower back if done incorrectly.

Pose 7: High Push-up

This pose is excellent for building upper body and core strength. It helps the lower back and allows for a lengthening of the spine. For a golfer, this is important as it builds strength to help with the arms and swinging muscles while building core strength to protect and lengthen the back.

Instructions:

1. From the Half-way Lift, place palms firmly on the ground spreading fingers widely apart.

2. Extend legs backward and get on toes.

3. Tuck the tailbone under so the legs, hips, and torso are in one straight line.

4. Extend the crown of your head forward.

5. Press your heels back.

6. Hold for 3–5 breaths. The longer you hold, the more strength you gain.

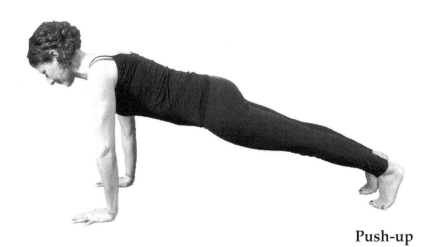

Push-up

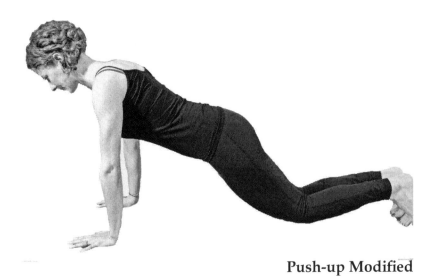

Push-up Modified

Position:

- Align your shoulder, elbows, and wrists so they are in one line.

- Use your core and your legs to hold this pose.

- Gently lift and engage your abdominal muscles.

- Your spine, legs, and neck should form one straight line.

Cautions:

If you have shoulder, arm or wrist injury, you can decrease the intensity by dropping your knees to the mat.

Contraindications:

Very tight hamstrings can lead to a pulled hamstring. Go very gently if you have tight hamstrings, and allow your body to warm up prior to going deeper into this exercise. Wrists can also be strained with this pose. Pressing down through the knuckles of your index fingers can relieve strain. Use your whole body to bring the force out of your wrists. If you move your thighbones back and engage them along with your core muscles, you will be able to remove some of the force from your wrists.

Pose 8: Low Push-up

The Low Push-up engages all of your muscles and can be very challenging at the beginning. It strengthens the upper and core body strength and if done correctly, will strengthen lower back muscles. The longer you hold this pose the more muscle strength you will build. Most people feel this in the arms too. This is a great pose for strengthening the muscles used in generating more swing speed.

Instructions:

1. From High Push-up, exhale and bend your elbows.

2. Move your body forward until your shoulders are at elbow height making a 90-degree angle at your elbow.

3. Tuck the tailbone under so the legs, hips, and torso are in one straight line.

4. Raise your chin slightly.

5. Press your heels back.

6. Hold for 3–5 breaths. The longer you hold, the more strength gains.

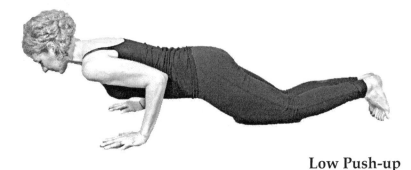

Low Push-up

Position:

- Align your elbows over your wrists and place them next to your ribs.

- The shoulders and elbows will form a straight line.

- Balance using the balls of your feet.

- Use your core and your legs to hold this pose.

- Gentle lift and engage your abdominal muscles.

- Your spine, legs, and neck should form one straight line.

- Remember to breathe.

Cautions:

If you have shoulder, arm, or wrist injury, you can decrease the intensity by dropping your knees to the mat. If that still isn't helping, drop your chest to the floor.

Contraindications:

Wrists can also be strained with this pose. Pressing down through the knuckles of your index fingers will minimize problems. Use your whole body to bring the force out of your wrists. If you move your thighbones back and engage them along with your core muscles, you will be able to remove some of the force from your wrists.

Pose 9: Downward Facing Dog

Instructions:

1. From Low Push-up pose, place your hands to the floor about shoulder width apart.

2. Start curling your toes back under your feet and press into the floor.

3. As you press with your toes, press with your hands and start walking your feet toward the back of the mat. Use your hips to lift your body. Keep your knees well bent.

4. Tilt your sit bones up to lengthen your spine.

5. Press down further attempting to place your heels to mat as well, although most people cannot do this.

6. Breathe deeply and freely.

7. Hold the pose for 3–6 breaths.

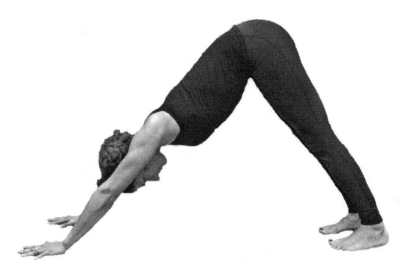

Downward Facing Dog

Position:

- Palms should be flat on the floor and fingers spread apart.

- Feel you thighs move back engaging your quad-riceps.

- Pull your navel towards your spine.

- Tilt your tailbone up.

- Drop your shoulder blades down your back and bring your elbows in.

- Bring your ears in line with your upper arms. This protects your neck while elongating the spine.

- Your feet should be hip width apart.

Cautions:

If your lower back is hurting intensely or you have pain, numbness, or tingling going down your leg, please visit your doctor immediately. While there may be tightness in the back, particularly in the lumbar region, that pain should be mild and under no circumstances should it radiate to another location below the back.

Contraindications:

Very tight hamstrings can lead to a pulled hamstring. Go very gently if you have tight hamstrings and allow your body to warm up prior to going deeper into this exercise.

Wrists can also be strained with this pose, so if they are troubling you, press down through the knuckles of your index fingers. Use your whole body to bring the force out of your wrists. Move your thighbones back and engage them along with your core muscles.

Pose 10: High Lunge

Also called the Crescent Pose, it helps the lower back and allows for a lengthening of the spine. High lunge is an excellent hip strengthener while stretching the muscles on the opposite side. For golfers, this allows for better range of motion and finish of the golf swing.

Instructions:

1. From Downward Facing Dog, exhale and step forward with your right foot between your hands aligning your knee over the heel. The left leg should be long and strong.

2. Inhale and raise the torso upright.

3. Bring your arms wide and raise them over your head with the palms facing one another.

4. Lengthen your tailbone towards the floor, reaching your left heel.

5. Hold for 4–8 breaths.

6. Exhale and release the torso to the right thigh.

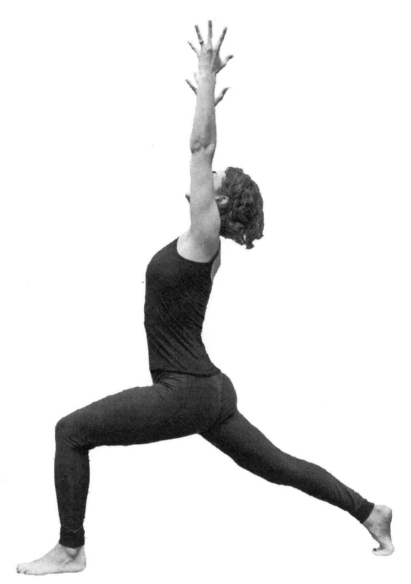

High Lunge

Position:

- Keep your back legs long and strong.

- Arms should be straight over your head with palms facing one another.

- Do not overarch the lower back.

- Bring the shoulder blades deep into the back to support the chest.

- Allow your ribs to drop to the floor.

Cautions:

People with high blood pressure or heart conditions may want to consult with a health professional prior to using this pose. Also it can provoke increased strain in the lower back region.

Pose 11: Warrior I

This pose stretches the chest, lungs shoulder, neck, belly, and groin while strengthening the thighs, calves, ankles, arms, shoulders, and back. Warrior allows for the hips to open as well. For golfers, this pose is invaluable as it helps with balance and strength of so many muscles groups.

Instructions:

1. From High Lunge, exhale and lunge forward with your right foot to create a 90-degree angle at the knee.

2. Spin your left (back) foot to a flat position at a 60-degree angle with your heels in one line.

3. Inhale and bring your hands over your head beside your ears, palms facing one another.

4. Hold for 30–60 seconds.

Position:

- Keep heels in one line.

- Square your hips bringing your right (forward) hip back.

- Engage your tailbone by scooping down and forward.

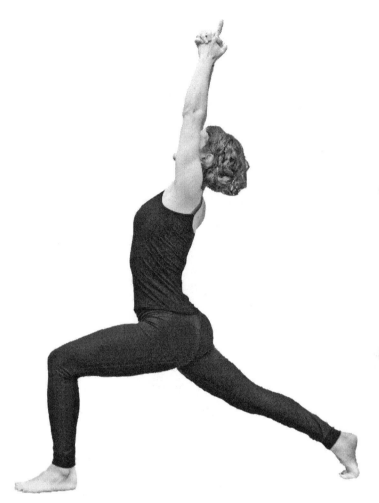

Warrior I

Cautions:

People with high blood pressure or heart conditions may want to consult with a health professional prior to using this pose. If you have shoulder issues, keep arms raised in slightly wider than parallel. If you have a neck problem, do not look up as this can put additional strain on your neck.

Pose 12: Rotating Crescent Lunge/Extending Side Angle

This is excellent for strengthening and stretching the legs, knees, and ankles. It also stretches the groin, spine, chest, lungs, and shoulders. It improves digestion and balance and increases stamina. For golfers, this pose increases balance and rotational stretching in the hips. This allows for improved turns on swings and the ability to generate more power through the swing without losing balance.

Instructions:

1. With your right foot forward in high lunge pose, rotate the torso, bringing the left elbow on the right knee.

2. Place the left hand on the ground on the outside of your right foot. You will need to turn your torso. Bring your palms together as if in prayer. Press into them to rotate the right shoulder up and back twisting the upper back.

3. Look at the wall or the ceiling.

4. Hold for 3–6 breathes.

5. To release: inhale and press into the feet, straightening the legs, and then inhale the arms out to the side or up towards the ceiling.

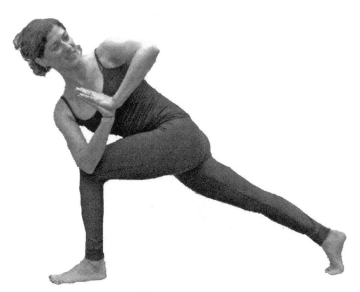

Crescent Lunge

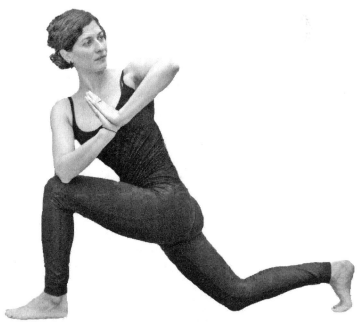

Crescent Lunge Modified

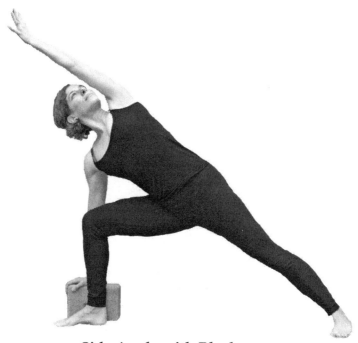

Side Angle with Block

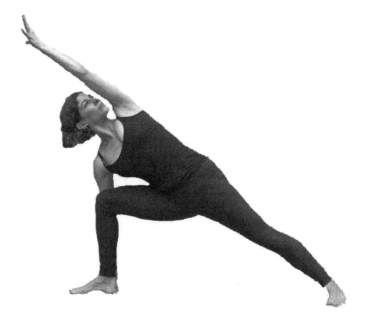

Side Angle with No Block

Position:

- Maintain your heels so they are in one line.

- Keep the outer edge of the back foot pressed into the mat.

- Keep you back leg very straight.

- Stack your torso on top of your right thigh.

Modifications:

If you can't put your foot flat on the floor, do the best you can.

Contraindications:

Don't do this if you have high or low blood pressure, and a headache. If you have neck problems or back injury, this could be a pose that can be harmful. With a neck injury, don't twist your neck at the end.

Pose 13: Low Lunge

This pose works in the thigh and groin regions. It helps the lower back and allows for a lengthening of the spine. This opens up the hips to allow for better rotation and balance in one's golf swing.

Instructions:

1. Exhale and place your hands back on mat.

2. Lower your back knee to the mat and place back foot flat on mat.

3. Place hands on your front knee and breathe deeply as you stretch your inner groin on the left and your thigh on the right.

4. Keep your chest high and bring your arms up towards the ceiling.

5. Hold for 5 breaths.

Position:

*   Maintain length in your spine and keep your chest up.

*   Tuck your tailbone under and lift your pubic bone under to improve balance.

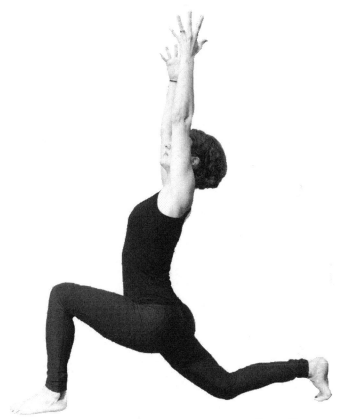

Low Lunge

- Practice this pose facing a wall. Press the big toe of the front foot against the wall and stretch your arms up, fingertips to the wall.

Contraindications:

This stretches the thigh greatly and if you have problems with your knees, it can cause problems.

Pose 14: One-Legged Pigeon

This pose allows you to stretch the entire front of the torso, the ankles, thighs, groins, abdomen, and chest. The quadriceps and psoas muscles are where you will feel the most. It is helpful for improving posture and alignment of the neck and chest.

Instructions:

1. Bring your back knee down to the floor.

2. Bring both hands to your front knee.

3. Reach back with your left hand and grab your back foot.

4. Pull your foot towards your buttock.

5. Stay for 5 breaths.

Position:

*   The intensity can be increased or decreased by leaning forward.

*   Leaning forward and pulling the back leg back further will increase intensity on the psoas.

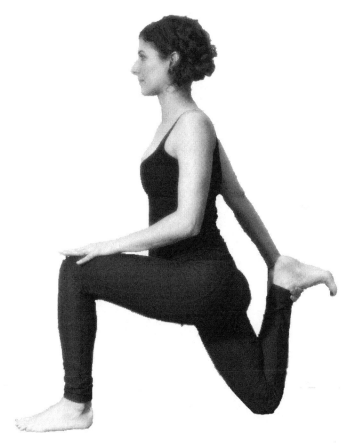

One-legged Pigeon

Cautions:

Do not lean on your kneecap! You want to position the back leg in such a way that the bottom of the thighbone is what contacts the floor. If you have knee issues, do this pose very carefully.

Pose 15: Half Pigeon

This pose opens the hips and chest. It is an excellent pose to stretch the thighs, hips, groin, psoas, and abdomen. It can be an extremely intense pose for many people, so please be sure to look at the modifications that can be made to help. This is another pose to help release tightness in the hips. This tightness can lead to an inability to turn properly increases slices and fades as your hips don't rotate properly.

Instructions:

1. Place your hands on the mat on either side of your front knee.

2. Slide the back leg back, lowering the hips towards the floor.

3. Press down into the palms or fingertips placed near your hips, inhale and reach with the top of your head, lengthening the spine. Exhale and bring the hips down to the floor. Roll the shoulders down and back. Lean forward through the chest.

4. Move as deep into the posture as you can while still maintaining full deep breathing.

5. Breathe and hold for 3–6 breaths.

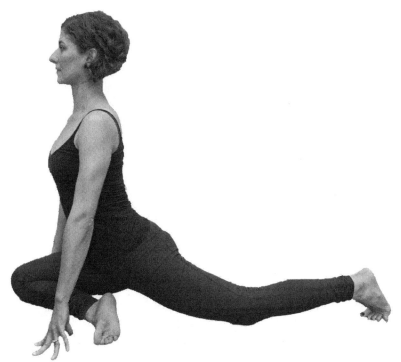

Half Pigeon

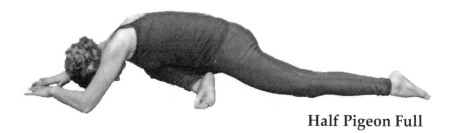

Half Pigeon Full

Position:

- The left leg should be straight back and not be angled to the side. It will rotate in slightly. Hold your foot up. Leaning forward puts more stretch into the thigh. Placing the back knee further back stretches psoas that goes up to the front of the abdomen.

- Place a folded blanket underneath the hip of the bent knee to keep the hips level. Use yoga blocks under the hands.

- Adjust the level of stretch in the hips by how close the foot of the bent knee is to the hips; bring it closer to the hips for less stretch, slide it away for more stretch.

- Any or all of these can be added to the treatment.

Cautions:

If you have knee, ankle, or sacroiliac injuries, please consult your healthcare provider as to the safety of this pose. Tight hips or thighs will make this pose difficult and uncomfortable but could be useful once warmed up.

Pose 16: Boat Pose

This pose is an excellent one to build abdominal muscles, hip flexors, and spine. It improves balance. It also helps stretch one's hamstrings. Overall this pose is most effective for helping build the muscles in the abdomen.

Instructions:

1. Sit on the floor with your legs straight. Keep your hands on the floor a little behind your hips.

2. Lift you chest up from the sternum and lean back slightly without rounding your back. Sit on the place between your sit bones.

3. Exhale, bend your knees and lift your feet off the floor with thighs angled about 45 degrees relative to the floor. Lift your pubis toward your navel and if you can, straighten your knees.

4. Raise your toes to about eye level, or if you can't, straighten your legs bring your shins parallel to the floor

5. Stretch your arms alongside your legs parallel to the floor. Bring your shoulder blades back and reach with your fingers.

6. Hold for 3–5 breaths and try to increase the time to 1 minute. Release on exhale and return to the sitting position.

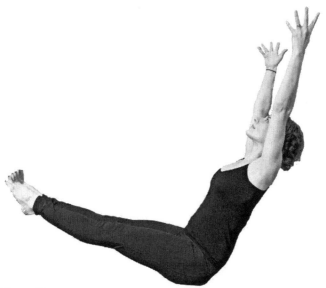

Boat Pose

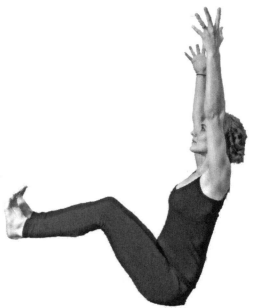

Boat Pose Modified

Position:

- Ensure your arms are parallel to the floor.

- Use your thighs to anchor the pose.

- While the belly should be firm it should not be hard or thick. Try to keep it flat.

Modifications:

If you cannot do the full pose, do the half pose by bringing your legs up with knees and feet at 90-degree angle. Clasp your hands around the back of your knees.

Contraindications:

Recent or chronic injury to the abdomen, knees, hips, arms, or shoulders.

If you have issues with your heart or low blood pressure, this is probably not a good pose without consulting a physician. If you are pregnant, you also may want to consult your doctor.

If you have a neck injury, sit with your back near a wall and rest your head against the wall to relieve the pressure in your neck.

Pose 17: Half Lord of Fishes

This is a great pose for cleansing the liver, kidneys, and stimulating digestion. It can help when one has a backache. It can be very useful for stretching the shoulders, hips, and neck while lengthening and opening the spine. For golfers, this pose is invaluable! I use this pose sometimes during a round if my back tightens. It stretches the area of the lower back that tends to ache in many golfers during or after a round. As golf is a one-way sport, the muscles on one side of the back sometimes get overused relative to the other. This creates issues due to the imbalance. This pose helps stretch the tight areas and strengthen the weaker ones.

Instructions:

1. Bring your legs down to the floor. You can use a blanket to support your bottom.

2. Bend your knees and put feet on the floor.

3. Slide your left foot under your right leg to the side of the hip and place the right foot over the left leg with the knee pointing up.

4. Exhale and twist towards the right thigh.

5. Press the right hand against the floor behind you and place the left upper arm on the outside of the right thigh near the knee.

6. Pull your torso up, press the right inner foot into the floor and release the right groin.

7. Breathe for 30–60 seconds, raising the sternum up each time. You can increase the stretch by twisting a little more each time.

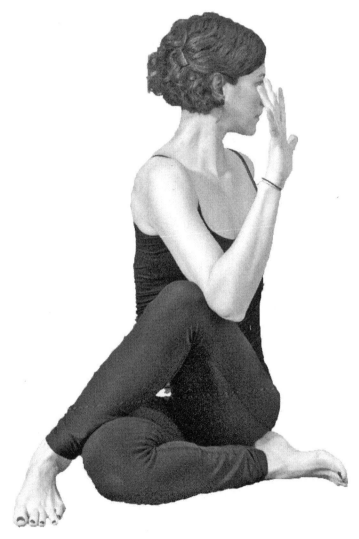

Half Lord of Fishes

Position:

- Keep the sternum straight up.

- The foot with the bent knee should be active and planted to the floor.

- Engage your tailbone by lengthening into the floor.

Cautions/Modifications:

A yoga block or folded blanket under the floor can help relieve any pressure.

Be sure not to over stretch your back.

Pose 18: Seated Forward Bend

This pose stretches the spine, shoulders, and hamstrings. It helps calm the brain and relieve depression. It can help improve digestion. It also continues the stretch started with the standing forward bend, but with slightly different angles of the muscles.

Instructions:

1. Straighten your legs in front of you so they are together with the ankles touching.

2. Use your hands to pull your sitting muscles out laterally so you come right onto your sitting bones.

3. Reach forward from your hips to grab your feet, ankles, or legs with both hands.

4. Inhale and flatten your back.

5. Exhale and fold forward.

6. Hold for 30–60 seconds.

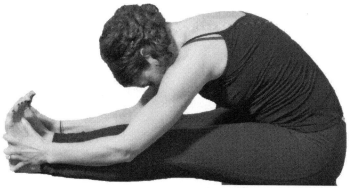

Seated Forward Bend

Position:

- Flex your feet.

- Hinge at your hips and not at your waste.

- Press your thighs toward the floor.

- Rotate your thighs downward.

- Allow your neck to be in neutral position.

Modifications/Cautions:

- You can use a yoga strap around your feet and hold on to the strap with your hands.

- Bend the knees enough to reach the feet with the hands and to place the head on the knees.

- Don't overstretch.

- If you have sciatica or recent lower back injury, check with your healthcare provider prior to doing this pose.

Pose 19: Dead Bug

This pose is excellent for stretching your groin, hips, and spine. It calms the brain and can be helpful for relieving stress and fatigue. This pose also helps create more flexion in the lower back, which can tighten. By lengthening this area, the rest of the back is less likely to tighten.

Instructions:

1. Lie on your back. Exhale and bend knees towards belly.

2. Inhale and grab the outsides of your feet with hands.

3. Open the knees slightly wider than torso to bring towards armpits.

4. Flex through heels aligning ankles over knees so shins are perpendicular to the floor.

5. Bring thighs closer to the torso to length your spine. Release the tailbone towards the floor and length your head away from the spine.

6. Hold for 30–60 seconds, and then release.

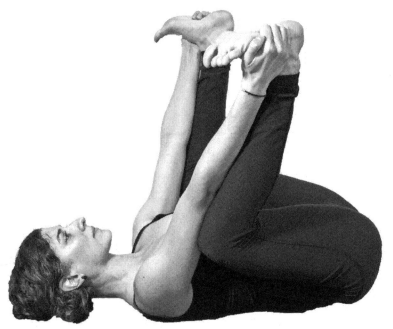

Dead Bug

Position:

- Keep ankles and knees in alignment.

- You can bring knees into chest for a reduced.

Modifications:

Use a belt or yoga strap to hold your feet in position if you can't reach.

Cautions:

Don't do this pose if you have a knee injury, neck injury, or are pregnant.

Pose 20: Corpse Pose

Savasana or the Corpse pose is essential to practice at the end of every yoga practice. This posture rejuvenates the body, mind, and spirit while reducing stress and tension. Corpse pose is meant to be a time to let go. It is a gathering of energy to move forward with your day.

Instructions:

1. Lying on your back, let the arms and legs drop open, with the arms about 45 degrees from the side of your body. Make sure you are warm and comfortable; if you need to, place blankets under or over your body. You can also use bolsters or blankets under knees if your lower back is a problem.

2. Close your eyes and breathe slowly and deeply through the nose. Allow your entire body to become soft and heavy, letting it relax into the floor. As the body relaxes, feel your body rise and fall with each breath.

3. In your mind's eye, scan the body from the toes to the fingers to the crown of the head, looking for tension, lightness and contracted muscles. Allow the release of this tension. You may find it better to move that part of the body or contract the muscles in the area to effect a release.

4. Release all control of the breath, the mind, and the body. Let your body move deeper and deeper into a state of total relaxation.

5. Stay in Savasana for 5–15 minutes.

6. To release: slowly deepen the breath, wiggle the fingers and toes, reach the arms over your head and stretch the whole body, then exhale, bend the knees into the chest, and roll over to one side coming into a fetal position. When you are ready, slowly inhale up to a seated position.

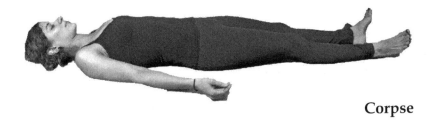

Corpse

Cautions:

If you have a back injury or discomfort, you can do the pose with your feet on the floor. A bolster under the lower back sometimes helps to relieve the pressure as well.

Week 2: Sitting Sequence

This sequence is excellent for gaining focus and strength while stretching the body. Generally this sequence should be used at a time that is not at the golf course. One could do this prior to playing or on a non-golf day. Used prior to play, it is an excellent way to gain mental focus for the day's match. Use it to quiet your mind and stay focused on breath. On other days or other times, it is important to focus on the stretch, and the strength building aspects of each pose. Balancing Table and Tiger are particularly important for one's swing as they help not only strengthen the core but work on gaining more balance.

Pose 1: Easy Pose

This is a calming pose that strengthens the back while stretching the knees and ankles. It helps the upper and lower back and is the familiar pose used in meditation. Some people will feel this more in their thighs than knees or back. This not only stretches the back, but also allows for strengthening. This strengthening is vital for a good golf swing as it strengthens the areas that are used to rotate during a swing.

Instructions:

1. If needed, fold a blanket or use a pillow to sit on. Six inches in height should help relieve some of the pressure. Sit close to the edge of this support with your legs in front of you.

2. Cross your shins, slipping each foot beneath the opposite knee while bending your knees towards your torso.

3. Slip the arches of each foot under the opposite shin, allowing your knees to widen.

4. Press your hands into the floor to lift your sit bones slightly. Make your thighbones heavy and then lower your self back to the floor. This should allow for the pelvis to be in neutral.

5. Place your hands on your lap or knees with palms.

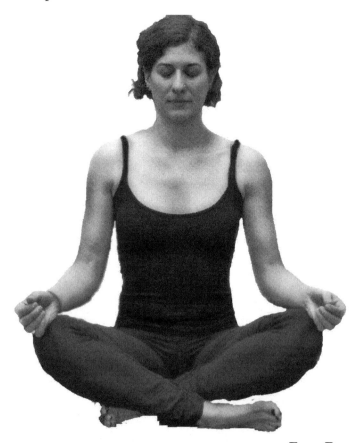

Easy Pose

Position:

- Allow the outer edges of your feet to rest comfortably on the floor.

- You should form a triangle amongst your two thighs and folded shins.

- Your pelvis should be in a relatively neutral position.

Cautions:

If you have knee problems or lower back injury, speak to a healthcare provider about doing this pose.

Pose 2: Cat-Cow

Instructions:

1. Come down unto hands and knees as if you are going to crawl.

2. While inhaling, tilt your sit bones up towards the sky. Draw your shoulder blades down your back and lift your gaze.

3. Exhale and round your spine towards the ceiling while lifting your navel (belly-button) towards your spine.

4. Do this 3–5 times.

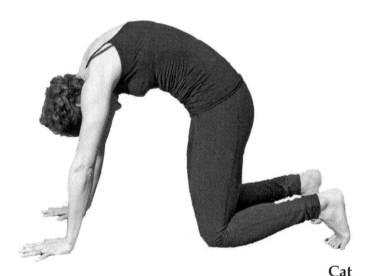

Cat

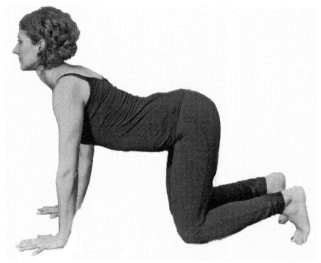

Cow

Position:

- Keep your hands under your shoulders and parallel to each other.

- Your knees should be shoulder width apart with your thighs perpendicular to the floor.

- While rounding your back go slowly and notice the tight areas. Those are the ones that you want to lengthen so that they get a complete stretch.

- Most golfers will feel cat in their lumbar region as they round the spine. By trying to lengthen that region a greater stretch will occur. Go easy though as if you stretch too much, too fast, you can hurt your back.

- You can also take several breaths in each position while lengthening your body. This deepens the stretch.

Cautions:

If your lower back is hurting intensely or you have pain, numbness, or tingling going down your leg, please visit your doctor immediately. While there may be tightness in the back, particularly in the lumbar region, that pain should be mild and under no circumstances should it radiate to another location below the back.

Recent or chronic injury to knees, shoulders or neck could make this pose difficult. Please consult with your clinician if this is the case.

Pose 3: Thread the Needle

Instructions:

1. From the above starting position, slide your left arm under your right, creating a bridge with your right arm.

2. Bring your right arm forward and form a 90-degree angle at the elbow.

3. Continue to slide your left arm under until you are resting both your left ear and your left shoulder on the mat.

4. Find the position where you feel the deepest stretch.

5. Hold the pose for 3–6 breaths and then do the other side.

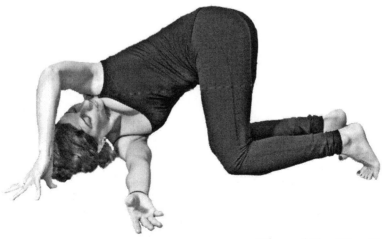

Thread the Needle

Position:

- Keep your shoulder and ear to the ground.

- Keep the non-threaded arm at a 90-degree hinge at the elbow. That arm will appear to be in front of you.

- Breathe gently as you do this.

Modifications:

Place a folded blanket under the knees to protect them from stress and pressure. Cross the upper hand over the back and hold onto the inside of the opposite thigh. This can generate more stretch.

Contraindications:

Recent or chronic injury to the knees, shoulders, or neck can be exacerbated by this pose.

Pose 4: Child's Pose

Instructions:

1. From the Cat-Cow starting position, exhale and lower your hips towards your heels, insuring that your feet are flat on the floor.

2. Spread your knees apart slightly.

3. Extend your hands over your head while you bring your head down to the floor.

4. Hold the pose for 3–6 breaths.

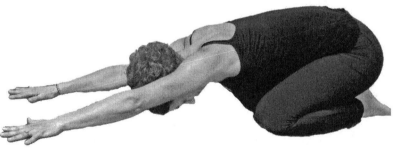

Child's Pose

Position:

- You should feel this in your lower back and your hips.

- Keep breathing into your belly as much as possible. This opens up the back and the sides.

- If your feet cramp, you can curl them such that the toes are under the floor.

- Keep your knees apart and your toes touching as if you are creating a V-shape with your legs.

Cautions:

If your lower back is hurting intensely or you have pain, numbness, or tingling going down your leg, please visit your doctor immediately. While there may be tightness in the back particularly in the lumbar region, that pain should be mild and under no circumstances should it radiate to another location below the back.

Contraindications:

Recent or chronic injury to knees, shoulders or neck could make this pose difficult. Please consult with your clinician if this is the case.

Pose 5: Downward Facing Dog

Instructions:

1. From Child's pose, place your hands to the floor about shoulder width apart.

2. Start curling your toes back under your feet and press into the floor.

3. As you press with your toes, press with your hands and start walking your feet toward the back of the mat. Use your hips to lift your body. Keep your knees well bent.

4. Tilt your sit bones up to lengthen your spine.

5. Press down further attempting to place your heels to mat as well, although most people cannot do this.

6. Breathe deeply and freely.

7. Hold the pose for 3–6 breaths.

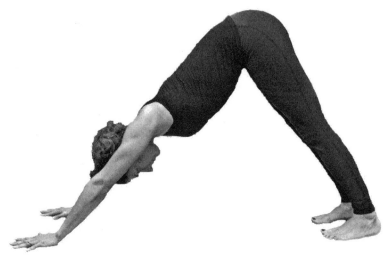

Downward Facing Dog

Position:

- Palms should be flat on the floor and fingers spread apart.

- Feel you thighs move back engaging your quadriceps.

- Pull your navel towards your spine.

- Tilt your tailbone up.

- Drop your shoulder blades down your back and bring your elbows in.

- Bring your ears in line with your upper arms. This protects your neck while elongating the spine.

- Your feet should be hip width apart.

Cautions:

If your lower back is hurting intensely or you have pain, numbness, or tingling going down your leg, please visit your doctor immediately. While there may be tightness in the back, particularly in the lumbar region, that pain should be mild and under no circumstances should it radiate to another location below the back.

Contraindications:

Very tight hamstrings can lead to a pulled hamstring. Go very gently if you have tight hamstrings and allow your body to warm up prior to going deeper into this exercise.

Wrists can also be strained with this pose, so if they are troubling you, press down through the knuckles of your index fingers. Use your whole body to bring the force out of your wrists. Move your thighbones back and engage them along with your core muscles.

Pose 6: Balancing Table

This pose is excellent for improving balance through building core-strength. It is very good for lengthening the spine and requires more strength than would first appear. Core strength exercises are very important for balance and protecting one's back.

Instructions:

1. Begin on your hands and knees placing your hands directly under your shoulders and your knees under your hips. (This is called Table pose.) Press the tops of your feet against the floor by uncurling your toes.

2. Align your head with your spine by fixing your gaze to a point between your palms.

3. Engage your abdominal muscles by pulling your belly button towards your spine without arching your back. Using your pelvic floor muscles, extend your right leg behind you. Flex your foot so that your toes point down and lengthen your legs while keeping your spine neutral.

4. Extend your left arm forward to shoulder height reaching out with your fingertips and lift your right leg off the floor to hip level.

5. Hold for 3–5 breaths.

6. Exhale and come back to Table pose.

7. Repeat on the other side extending the right arm and the left leg. Hold for the same amount of time.

8. Repeat 5–10 times.

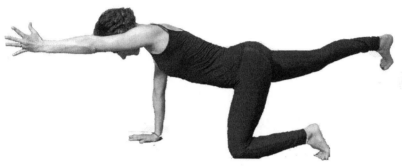

Balancing Table

Position:

- Ensure that your hips are above the knees and that hands are below shoulders.

- Make sure both your lifted arm and leg are fully extended.

- Keep the extended limbs at the correct level.

Modifications/Cautions:

- A mat or blanket under knees can relieve pressure.

- If you have a wrist issue, you can balance on your fist to relieve the pressure to the wrist.

Contraindications:

Do not practice this pose if you have recent or chronic injury to the knee, arms, wrists, shoulders or back.

Pose 7: Tiger Pose

This pose warms and stretches the back muscles and spine. Tiger allows for a gentle stretching of the lower back and strengthening of the gluteal muscles. This is a great pose to do prior to leaving for a round of golf, as it gets the blood flowing and the body moving.

Instructions:

1. Place your hands and knees on the floor as you did at the start of Balancing Table position.

2. Inhale and bring the right knee to the forehead, rounding the spine.

3. Exhale and bring the right foot up towards the ceiling, arching the spine, and looking up at the ceiling.

4. Ensure that you have engaged your pelvic floor muscles as you bring the leg back and over your head.

5. Repeat this 4–8 times.

6. Repeat on other side.

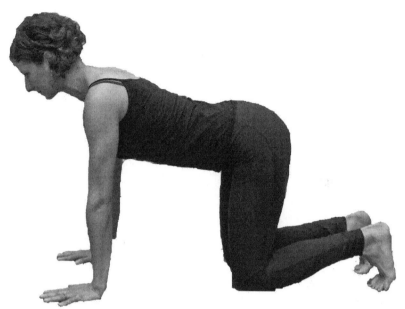

Start

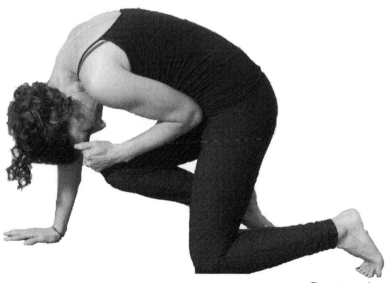

Contraction

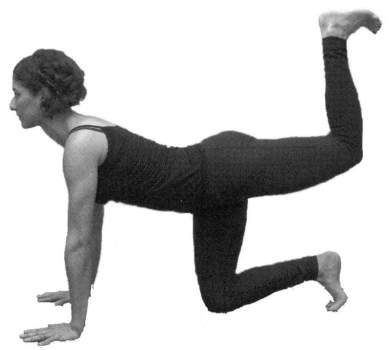

Expansion

Position:

- Perform this slowly and keep the knee in alignment.

- You can also lift your leg and hold it.

- Use a blanket or mat under your knees if there is too much pressure on them.

Cautions:

Recent or chronic injury to the back, hips, or knees.

Pose 8: Locust

This pose is sometimes called Superman pose as you lay on your stomach and lift your arms and legs up as if flying through the air. It strengthens the spine, buttocks, and backs of the arms and legs. It stretches the front of the body including shoulders, chest, belly, and thighs. It improves posture, stimulates digestion, and helps relieve stress. For golfers, this is another pose that is excellent for strengthening the areas used in the rotation of a swing. The lower back muscles tend to fatigue if not worked, and locust pose improves this strength.

Instructions:

1. Lie on your belly with chin on the floor and legs together and arms alongside the body. Turn your big toes toward each other to rotate the thighs inward. Firm buttocks pressing your coccyx towards your pubis.

2. Exhale and lift head, upper torso, arms, and legs away from the floor. This causes you to rest on your lower ribs, belly, and front pelvis. (You may want to use a blanket under any parts that are sore.) Keep the big toes turned towards each other.

3. Raise your arms parallel to the floor to stretch back. Press scapulas into your back.

4. Breathe and hold for 3–6 breaths (up to one minute).

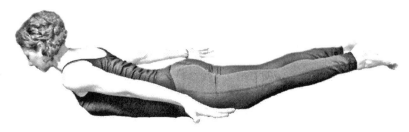

Locust

Position:

- Start with arms 45 degrees away from the sides, with the palms down.

- Turn your big toes toward each other to rotate the thighs inward.

- Keep the neck in line with the spine pulling through the top of your head towards the wall in front.

Modifications:

- Place a folded blanket under the pelvis or place a rolled up blanket or bolster under the thighs.

- Place a rolled blanket under the rib cage.

- To strengthen your lower back, bring the arms out to the sides or forward over your head.

Contraindications:

Recent or chronic injury to the back, arms, or shoulders, pregnancy, menstruation, or recent abdominal surgery could cause serious problems. Check with your healthcare provider about doing this pose with these issues or serious neck injury.

Pose 9: Sphinx Pose

This pose stretches the chest and lungs, shoulders and abdomen, firms the buttocks, and strengthens the spine. For golfers, this pose is excellent for stretching the upper back and neck.

Instructions:

1. Lie on your belly with tailbone towards your pubis. Lengthen towards your heel.

2. Rotate your thighs inwardly by rolling your outer thighs toward the floor to broaden and lengthen your back and sacrum.

3. Reach with your toes behind you.

4. Press your forearms down into the floor and inhale and lift the head and chest off the floor. Keep your elbows under your shoulders with forearms parallel to the floor.

5. Inhale and lift your upper torso and head from the floor into a mild backbend. Only go as far as is comfortable.

6. Hold for 5–10 breaths.

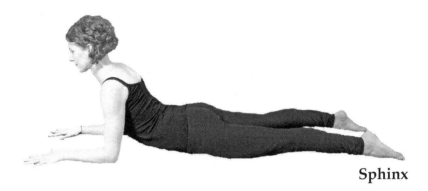

Sphinx

Position:

- Keep your abdomen engaged. You don't have to suck in your belly.

- Keep your elbows parallel.

Cautions:

Avoid if you have recent or chronic injury to the back, arms or shoulders, pregnancy or recent abdominal surgery.

Pose 10: Bow Pose

This is an excellent pose for stretching the entire front of the body, ankles, thighs, and groins. It opens the chest and abdomen. It is an excellent exercise to do if you perform many crunches because it will allow for a stretching of those muscles. It also improves posture by strengthening the back muscles.

Instructions:

1. Lie on your belly with your hands beside your torso with your palms up.

2. Exhale and bend knees bringing heels as close to buttocks as possible.

3. Grab your ankles with your hands.

4. Inhale and lift your heels away from your buttocks while lifting your thighs off the floor. Your head and torso should also lift from the floor as a result of this action.

5. Press shoulder blades against back to open chest and heart. Pull the tops of the shoulders away from your ears. Gaze forward.

6. Stay in pose for up to 30 seconds.

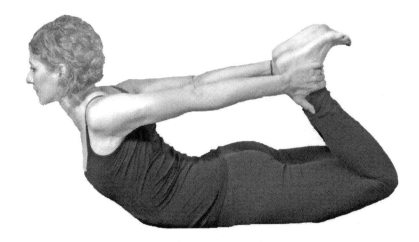

Bow

Position:

- Make sure your knees aren't wider than the width of your hips, and keep your knees hip width for the duration of the pose.

- Tilt your pelvis so that your tailbone points towards the floor.

- Soften the muscles in your back.

Modifications/Cautions:

- Some beginners may need to use a strap to reach their legs. A rolled up blanket can be used under the thighs to make easier.

- Consult with your healthcare provider if you have neck or lower-back injury.

Pose 11: Bridge Pose

This pose is excellent for stretching the chest, neck, and spine. It rejuvenates tired legs and helps alleviate stress. It can help with mild back pain. It can be a great pose to do after a round or workout to relieve tightness in the back.

Instructions:

1. Lie on your back with knees bent and feet flat on floor.

2. Place heels as close to your sit bones as possible.

3. Exhale and press your inner feet and arms into the floor. Push your tailbone upward towards your pubis.

4. Clasp your hands and lift your buttocks up until the thighs are parallel to the floor.

5. Lift your chin away from the sternum and press shoulder blades back.

6. Broaden your shoulders and lift the space between them and the base of your neck.

7. Hold for 30–60 seconds and release on exhalation.

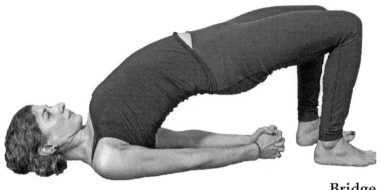

Bridge

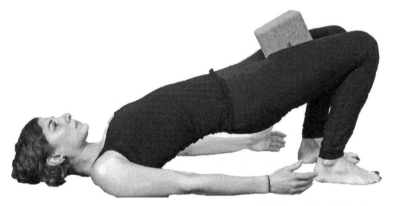

Bridge Modified

Position:

- Keep your thighs and feet parallel.

- Clasp the hands below your pelvis and extend through the arms to help you stay on the tops of your shoulders.

- To avoid over-stretching the neck, don't pull the shoulders forcefully away from the ears.

Cautions:

Neck injury can occur if done improperly. Also check with your healthcare provider if you have an existing injury.

Pose 12: Dead Bug

Instructions:

1. Release your position so you return to lying on your back.

2. Inhale and grab the outsides of your feet with your hands.

3. Open the knees slightly wider than torso to bring towards armpits.

4. Flex through heels aligning ankles over knees so shins are perpendicular to the floor.

5. Bring the thighs closer to the torso to lengthen your spine. Release the tailbone towards the floor and lengthen your head away from the spine.

6. Hold for 30–60 seconds, and then release.

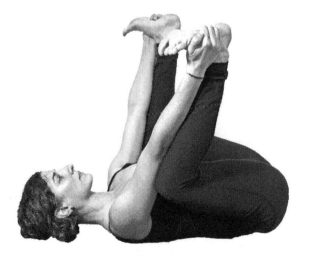

Dead Bug

Position

- Keep your ankles and knees in alignment.

- You can bring your knees into the chest.

- You can use a belt to assist you better if you cannot properly reach your feet at first.

Cautions

Check with your healthcare provider about doing if you have neck or knee injury.

Pose 13: Bound Angle Pose

This is an excellent pose to stretch the inner thighs and knees. It opens the pelvis and when done properly it will begin to open the back as well. It can be used to improve sciatica in some cases.

Instructions

1. Sit on the floor with your legs in front of you. Exhale and bend your needs pulling your heels into your pelvis. Allow your knees to drop to the sides and press your soles together.

2. Bring your heels towards your pelvis as comfortably as you can. Keep the outer edges of the feet together.

3. Sit so that the pubis in front and the tailbone in back are the same distance to the floor. The pelvis should be in a neutral position.

4. Lengthen your torso through the sternum.

5. Stay in this pose for 1–5 minutes while continuing to breathe.

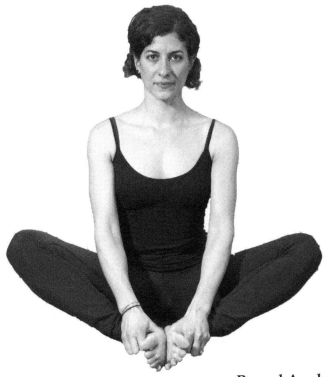

Bound Angle

Position:

- Do not force the knees done but rather allow the thigh ones to fall towards the floor.

- If your hips or groins are tight, use a blanket under your pelvis to lift.

Pose 14: Single Leg Scissors (Both Sides)

This pose is excellent for building abdominal and core muscle strength. What's great about this pose is that it engages the entire body to coordinate movements; something that is similar when performing a golf swing.

Instructions:

1. Lay on the floor flat and then bring your knees to your chest.

2. Place your hands behind your head and extend your legs to the ceiling.

3. Lower one leg down to about 6–12 inches above the floor

4. Keeping your legs strong, flex your feet and lift your head and shoulders off the floor

5. While breathing as fully as possible, engage your stomach muscles and pull your torso up

6. Hold for 10 counts

7. Reverse legs and do the other side.

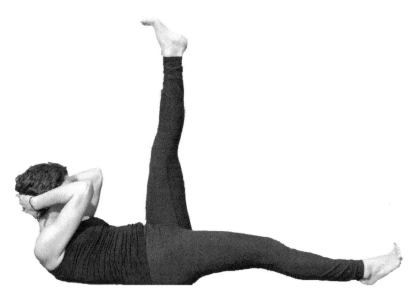

Scissors

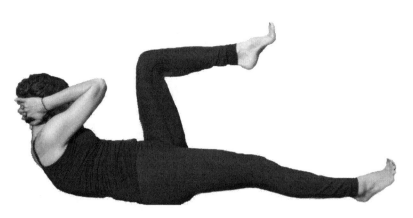

Scissors Modified

Position:

- Be sure to keep your abdominal muscles engaged as not doing so may cause lower back pain.

Modifications/Cautions

- If you feel strain in your lower back, place the leg that is up in the air down on the ground with your sole flat on it and knee bent.

- If you cannot keep your leg straight in the air due to tight hamstrings, ensure that your knee is pointing up to the ceiling straight and bend the lower half of your leg

Pose 15: Boat Pose

This pose is an excellent one to build abdominal muscles, hip flexors, and spine. It improves the balance. It also helps stretch one's hamstrings. Overall this pose is most effective for helping you build abdominal muscles. This extra core strength helps generate power in one's swing.

Instructions:

1. Sit on the floor with legs straight. Keep your hands on the floor a little behind your hips.

2. Lift your chest up from the sternum and lean back slightly without rounding your back. Sit on the place between your sit bones.

3. Exhale, bend your knees and lift your feet off the floor with thighs angled about 45 degrees relative to the floor. Lift your pubis toward your navel and if you can, straighten your knees.

4. Raise your toes to about eye level or if you can't straighten your legs, bring your shins parallel to the floor.

5. Stretch your arms alongside your legs parallel to the floor. Bring your shoulder blades back and reach with your fingers.

6. Hold for 3–5 breaths and try to increase time
    to 1 minute. Release on exhale and return to
    the sitting position.

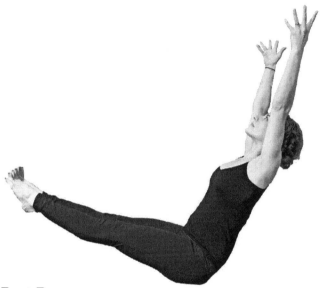

Boat Pose

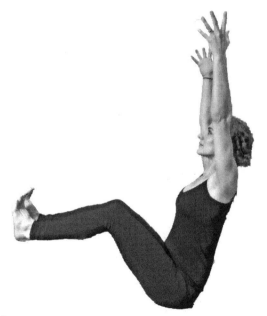

Boat Pose Modified

Position:

- Ensure your arms are parallel to the floor.

- Use your thighs to anchor the pose.

- While the belly should be firm it should not be hard or thick. Try to keep it flat.

Modifications/Cautions

- If you cannot do the full pose, do the half pose. This is performed by bringing your legs up with knees and feet at a 90-degree angle.

- Clasp your hands around the back of your knees.

- Recent or chronic injury to the abdomen, knees, hips, arms, or shoulders.

- If you have issues with your heart or low blood pressure, this is probably not a good pose without consulting a physician. If you are pregnant, you also may want to consult your doctor.

- If you have a neck injury, sit with your back near a wall and rest your head against the wall to relieve the pressure in your neck.

Pose 16: Seated Pigeon

This pose is a great pose to open the hips one at a time. It stretches the piriformis muscle, which tightens in golfers or people who sit a lot. With opening of the hips, your swing should be easier and smoother.

Instructions:

1. From the boat pose, bring your legs down in front of you with hands placed slightly behind you and to the sides.

2. Cross your right foot over the top of the thigh, keeping your shin parallel to the floor.

3. You can use your hands to walk your torso forward intensifying the stretch.

4. Hold for 5 breathes and you can repeat on the other side.

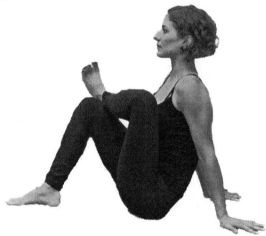

Seated Pigeon

Position:

- Keep your spine straight to lengthen.

- Keep your torso up

Cautions:

If you have a wrist injury, don't push too hard. Take care if you have a lower back injury.

Pose 17: Half Backward Plank

This pose is a counter to the hip work. It opens things going the other way and allows for a relaxation of the muscles that were just stretched.

Instructions:

1. From Seated Half Pigeon, move your hands further back behind you.

2. Keeping your legs crossed; push up through your hands and your lower foot so that your hips lift into the air.

3. Align your head with your spine holding in the air.

4. Hold for 5 breaths and you can repeat on the other side.

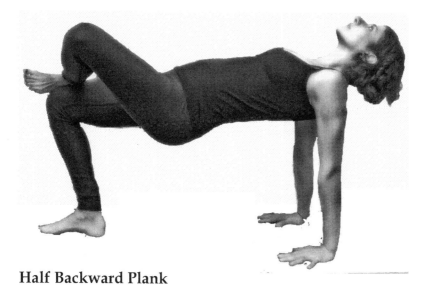

Half Backward Plank

Position:

- Move your shoulder blades towards each other.

- Keep your hips lifted as high as you can.

Cautions:

If you have a wrist injury, don't push too hard. Also take care if your neck is injured. You can simply release your neck so that your chin points to the ceiling.

Pose 18: Half Lord of Fishes

Instructions:

1. Bring your legs down to the floor. You can use a blanket to support your bottom.

2. Bend your knees and put feet on the floor.

3. Slide your left foot under your right leg to the side of the hip and place the right foot over the left leg with the knee pointing up.

4. Exhale and twist towards the right thigh.

5. Press the right hand against the floor behind you and place the left upper arm on the outside of the right thigh near the knee.

6. Pull your torso up, press the right inner foot into the floor and release the right groin.

7. Breathe for 30–60 seconds, raising the sternum up each time. You can increase the stretch by twisting a little more each time.

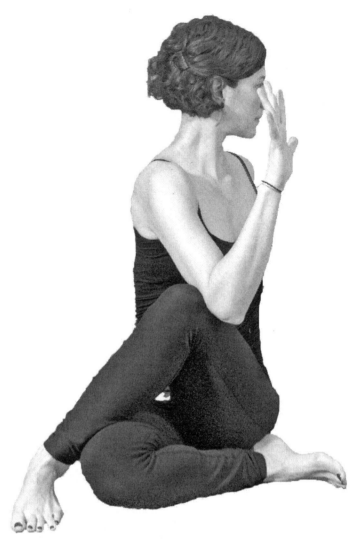

Half Lord of Fishes

Position:

- Keep the sternum straight up.

- The foot with the bent knee should be active and planted to the floor.

- Engage your tailbone by lengthening into the floor.

Cautions/Modifications:

A yoga block or folded blanket under the floor can help relieve any pressure.

Be sure not to over stretch your back.

Pose 19: Staff Pose

This pose strengthens the back muscles and stretches the shoulders and chest and improves posture. It realigns the spine and gently stretches the backs of the legs.

Instructions:

1. Sit on the mat with legs together and straight in front of you.

2. Place hands on floor next to your hips palms down.

3. Press thighs into floor.

4. Lift chest and press with palms.

5. Tilt your sacrum slightly towards pelvis.

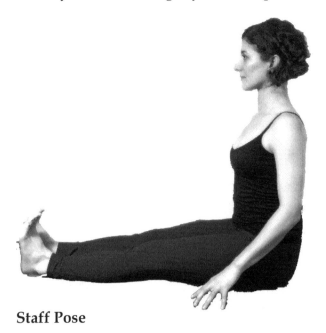

Staff Pose

Position:

- Press inner edges of feet forward.

- Keep your spine straight.

Cautions:

If you have a wrist injury, don't push too hard. Take care if you have a lower back injury.

Pose 20: Seated Forward Bend

Instructions:

1. Straighten your legs in front of you so they are together with the ankles touching.

2. Use your hands to pull your sitting muscles out laterally so you come right onto your sitting bones.

3. Reach forward from your hips to grab your feet, ankles, or legs with both hands.

4. Inhale and flatten your back.

5. Exhale and fold forward.

6. Hold for 30–60 seconds.

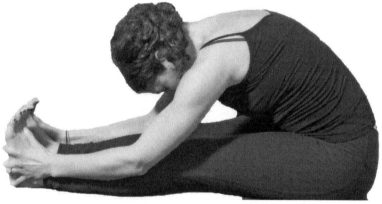

Seated Forward Bend

Position:

- Flex your feet.

- Hinge at your hips and not at your waste.

- Press your thighs toward the floor.

- Rotate your thighs downward.

- Allow your neck to be in neutral position.

Modifications/Cautions:

- You can use a yoga strap around your feet and hold on to the strap with your hands.

- Bend the knees enough to reach the feet with the hands and to place the head on the knees.

- Don't overstretch.

If you have sciatica or recent lower back injury, check with your healthcare provider prior to doing this pose.

Pose 21: Fish Pose

This is an excellent pose to stretch the psoas and the muscles between the ribs (intercostals). It also stretches the abdominal muscles and the front of the neck and upper back muscles. This is an excellent pose to improve posture. This helps improve breathing. For golfers, it also stretches the back muscles in the lower back.

Instructions:

1. Lower yourself to the floor slowly so that you are flat on your back with knees bent and feet flat on floor.

2. While inhaling, lift your pelvis slightly of the floor and slide your hands below your buttocks with your palms down.

3. Rest your buttocks on the backs of your hands and exhale.

4. Inhale and press your forearms and elbows firmly against the floor.

5. Press your scapulas into your back and lift your torso and head away from the floor.

6. Arch your back lifting your chest off the floor, resting your head on the floor.

7. Straighten your legs out onto the floor, keeping your thighs active, and press through your heels.

8. Stay in the position for 20–50 seconds. Exhale and lower your torso and head to the floor.

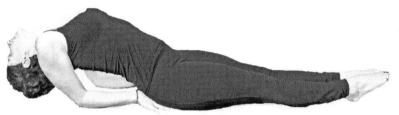

Fish Pose

Position:

- Ensure that you don't put too much weight on the floor as that can injure your neck.

- Be sure to tuck your forearms and elbows up close to the sides of your torso.

Modifications/Cautions:

This pose is very easy to strain your neck. If you feel any discomfort in your neck or throat, either lower the chest towards the floor until that subsides or place a folded blanket under the back of your head.

Pose 22: Hamstring Stretch

This pose stretches the hips, thighs, hamstrings, groin, and calves. It helps strengthen the knees and can help relieve mild back pain. Stretching the hamstrings may relieve sciatica. For golfers, hamstrings can tighten, and this tightness can affect your swing in many different ways. It decreases rotation and may increase lower back pain due to a transfer of muscle use to that area due to the stiffness in the hamstrings.

Instructions:

1. Lie flat on the floor with your legs fully extended.

2. Exhale and bend one knee towards your head.

3. Pull your thigh towards your belly and then press the other thigh into the floor.

4. Place a strap around the arch of your bent foot, holding the strap with both hands.

5. Inhale and straighten your knee pressing the heel up towards the ceiling.

6. Move your hands up the strap until your arms are fully extended. Press your shoulder blades gently into the floor.

7. Keep your raised leg fully extended. You can

alternate between pointing your toes to the ceiling and then flexing your foot.

8. Stay in the stretch for 2–3 minutes.

9. Extend the leg to the side swinging your leg out from the hip joint to the same side that the leg is on. You should feel the leg rotate and also feel the stretch more in your inner thigh.

10. Hold this position for 2–3 minutes as well.

11. Bring the leg back to the vertical stretch exhale and gently release the strap while bringing the leg back down to the floor.

12. Repeat on other side.

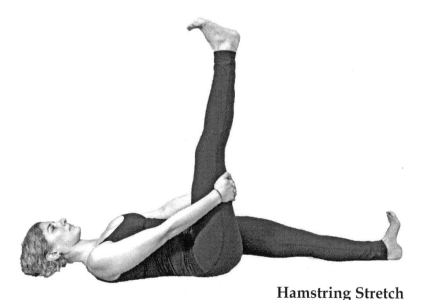

Hamstring Stretch

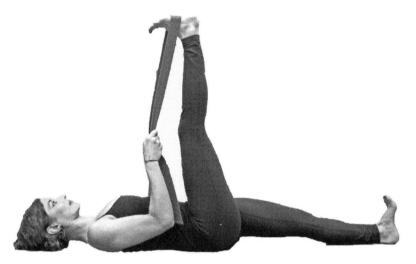

Hamstring Strap

Position

- If your head isn't comfortable, place a folded blanket underneath it.

- Keep the shoulder blades broad and flat on the floor.

- Keep your hands as high on the strap as possible.

- Move the collarbones away from the sternum.

Modifications/Cautions:

If you are extremely tight in the hamstrings, do this stretch with the non-active foot flat on the floor.

Be sure not to overstretch.

Pose 23: Supine Belly Twist

This pose is excellent for opening the back muscles. Twists stretch muscles along the sides of the body, the rib cage, and chest. It helps open breathing and as with all twists help stimulate the abdominal organs. For golfers, this pose improves range of motion that mimics a golf swing. It can help balance you to the side you don't use as much, which helps prevent injuries.

Instructions:

1. Lie on your side with your knees bent and your thighs together. Keeps your arms together as well.

2. Stretch your top arm out to the side so that your shoulders are at a 90-degree angle and your palms are on the ground.

3. Walk your hands back about six inches, keeping your palms grounded, and your fingers facing forward toward your toes.

4. Keep both shoulders firmly grounded and feel broadness across your chest. Lift your head just slightly and turn your gaze to the opposite side of your knees,. Stay for 3–5 breaths.

5. Inhale and bring your gaze then arm back to center.

6. Pause for a breath or two before taking the twist in the opposite direction.

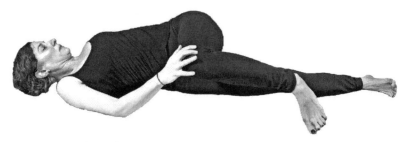

Supine Belly Twist

Position:

- Sometimes the shoulder on the opposite side of the body will lift when we twist. That is an indication that we have gone too far into the pose. Ease out a bit and be sure that both shoulders stay equally grounded.

- If needed, bring some support under your knees, either a blanket or block. As you progress, you may find that over time you no longer need the support and are able to release the knees all the way down while keeping the chest open and shoulders down.

Cautions:

Don't go too far or too fast. You can definitely overstretch yourself.

Pose 24: Corpse Pose

Instructions:

1. Lying on your back, let the arms and legs drop open, with the arms about 45 degrees from the side of your body. Make sure you are warm and comfortable; if you need to, place blankets under or over your body. You can also use bolsters or blankets under knees if your lower back is a problem.

2. Close your eyes and breathe slowly and deeply through the nose. Allow your entire body to become soft and heavy, letting it relax into the floor. As the body relaxes, feel your body rise and fall with each breath.

3. In your mind's eye, scan the body from the toes to the fingers to the crown of the head, looking for tension, tightness and contracted muscles. Allow the release of this tension. You may find it better to move that part of the body or contract the muscles in the area to effect a release.

4. Release all control of the breath, the mind, and the body. Let your body move deeper and deeper into a state of total relaxation.

5. Stay in Savasana for 5–15 minutes.

6. To release: slowly deepen the breath, wiggle the fingers and toes, reach the arms over your head and stretch the whole body, then exhale, bend the knees into the chest, and roll over to one side coming into a fetal position. When you are ready, slowly inhale up to a seated position.

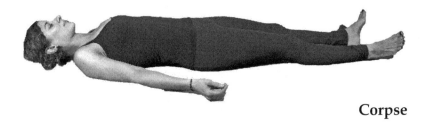

Corpse

Cautions:

If you have a back injury or discomfort, you can do the pose with your feet on the floor. A bolster under the lower back sometimes helps to relieve the pressure as well.

Week 3: Standing Only Sequence

This sequence is an excellent one to do prior to a round of golf. One can easily do this in a short amount of time. The idea is to use this as a warm-up prior to playing. It allows for the body to warm up gently and then gain some alignment prior to playing. Ensuring that your spine is aligned and the body is loose allows for one to flow more easily while one plays.

Pose 1: Mountain

This is a starting pose and is helpful for improving posture, firming the abdomen and buttocks and strengthening the thighs, knees, and ankles. It helps to lengthen the body.

Instructions:

1. Start by standing up straight. Drive your legs down while at the same time lifting your sternum up towards the ceiling. Imagine that you are stretching your feet and your head away from each other. Leave your hands down by your side, as if you are standing at attention.

2. Spin you palms outward, inhale and sweep your hands up sideways stopping when a shoulder's width apart above your head.

3. Lift your chin and gaze up at the ceiling.

4. Hold for 3–5 breaths.

Position:

- Reach your fingertips to the ceiling and root your feet into the floor.

- Keep your eyes focused on one point.

- Pull your stomach into your spine.

Cautions:

There are none for this pose.

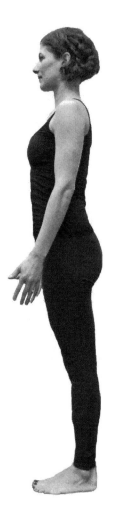

Mountain

Pose 2: Crescent Moon (to side)

This pose stretches and opens the sides of the body, which improves core strength and balance. It also strengthens the ankles and knees. I find this pose to be invaluable prior to playing golf. It somehow allows my hips to be more in alignment and gives me a full range of motion so that I can swing the club more easily. If you find yourself slicing or hooking the ball during a round consistently, it may be time to do this pose to help realign your body.

Instructions:

1. Bring your arms over your head and interlace fingers.

2. Press your feet into the floor and reach with your fingers and the tops of your head up while relaxing shoulders and back.

3. Exhale and press the right hip out to the side while arching over to the left. Keep your feet firmly planted and your buttocks engaged. Lengthen your arms and head.

4. Breathe and hold for 3–6 breathes.

5. Inhale and press your feet into the ground as you reach your fingers back to the ceiling.

6. Repeat the other side.

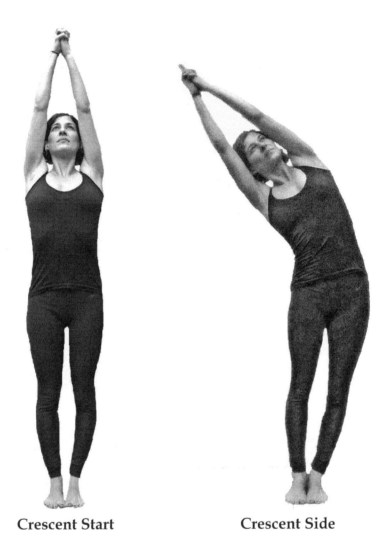

Crescent Start   **Crescent Side**

Position:

- Keep your feet planted firmly in the floor.

- Lift the hip on the opposite side slightly to lengthen the stretch on that side.

Modifications/Cautions:

- You can place your hand on the side that you are stretching towards on your hip for support and bring the other one over your head towards that side.

- Alternatively you could place the hand on the stretching side on your knee.

- Recent or chronic injury to the hips, back, or shoulders.

Pose 3: Chair

The Chair pose strengthens the lower body while stretching the upper back and chest. This posture invigorates and energizes the whole body. It strengthens the ankles, thighs, calves, and spine. This can help with flat feet.

1. From the Mountain pose inhale and raise your arms perpendicular to the floor.

2. Exhale and bend your knees into a squat. Reach back with your hips as if sitting on a chair. Keep your weight over your heels.

3. Press your shoulders down and back stretching between your shoulder blades, but without squeezing.

4. Breathe and hold for 3–6 breaths.

5. Release by inhaling and pressing down through the feet. Straighten your legs and inhale. Exhale while releasing arms.

Position:

- Keep arms straight up towards ceiling.

- Have your knees project out straight.

- Don't allow your thighs to get too parallel to the ground.

- Keep your tailbone pointing down to the floor.

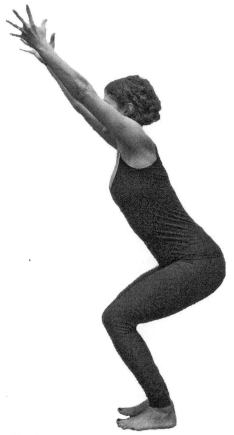

Chair

Modifications/Cautions:

- Placing hands on your knees will make this less challenging.

- To make more challenging and build thigh muscle faster, place a block between your thighs during the pose.

- Recent or chronic injury to the hips, knees, back, or shoulders.

Pose 4: Standing forward Bend

Instructions:

1. From Child's pose, place your hands to the floor about shoulder width apart.

2. Start curling your toes back under your feet and press into the floor.

3. As you press with your toes, press with your hands and start walking your feet toward the back of the mat.

4. Tilt your sit bones up to length your spine.

5. Press down further attempting to place your heels to mat as well although most people cannot do this.

6. Breathe deeply and freely.

7. Hold the pose for 3–6 breaths.

Position:

- Palms should be flat on the floor and fingers spread apart.

- Feel you thighs move back engaging your quadriceps.

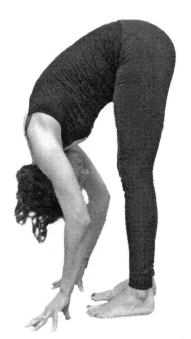

Standing Forward Bend

- Pull your navel towards your spine.

- Tilt your tailbone up.

- Slightly rotate your thighbones outward. (Move the front of your thigh away from your body.) This creates more strengthening of the pelvic floor.

- Drop your shoulder blades down your back and bring your elbows in.

Cautions:

If your lower back is hurting intensely or you have pain, numbness, or tingling going down your leg, please visit your doctor immediately. While there may be tightness in the back, particularly in the lumbar region, that pain should be mild and under no circumstances should it radiate to another location below the back.

Contraindications:

Very tight hamstrings can lead to a pulled hamstring. Go very gently if you have tight hamstrings and allow your body to warm up prior to going deeper into this exercise.

Wrists can also be strained with this pose so if they are troubling you, can pressing down through the knuckles of your index fingers. Use your whole body to bring the force out of your wrists. If you move your thighbones back and engage them along with your core muscles, you will be able to remove some of the force from your wrists.

Pose 5: Halfway lift

Instructions:

- From Standing Forward Bend, keep your feet to-gether and place your fingertips on the floor.

- Start curling your toes back under your feet and press into the floor.

- As you press with your toes, press with your hands and start walking your feet toward the back of the mat.

- Tilt your sit bones up to length your spine.

- Press down further attempting to place your heels to mat as well although most people cannot do this.

- Breathe deeply and freely.

- Hold the pose for 3–6 breaths.

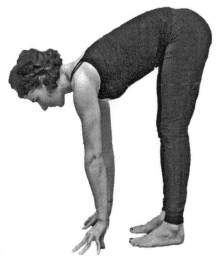

Halfway Lift

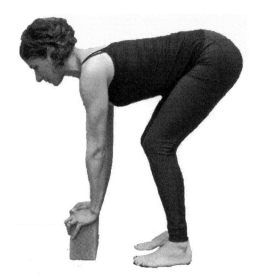

Halfway Lift Block

Position:

- Palms should be flat on the floor and fingers spread apart.

- Feel you thighs move back engaging your quadriceps.

- Pull your navel towards your spine.

- Tilt your tailbone up.

- Drop your shoulder blades down your back and bring your elbows in.

- Extend and lengthen your spine and bring your neck into alignment.

Cautions:

Very tight hamstrings can lead to a pulled hamstring. Go very gently if you have tight hamstrings and allow your body to warm up prior to going deeper into this exercise. Knees can be bent further to ensure a flat back.

Be careful if you've had a recent back injury because this can put a lot of pressure onto your lower back if done incorrectly.

Pose 6: Downward Facing Dog

Instructions:

1. From Child's pose, place your hands to the floor about shoulder width apart.

2. Start curling your toes back under your feet and press into the floor.

3. As you press with your toes, press with your hands and start walking your feet toward the back of the mat. Use your hips to lift your body. Keep your knees well bent.

4. Tilt your sit bones up to lengthen your spine.

5. Press down further attempting to place your heels to mat as well, although most people cannot do this.

6. Breathe deeply and freely.

7. Hold the pose for 3–6 breaths.

Position:

• Palms should be flat on the floor and fingers spread apart.

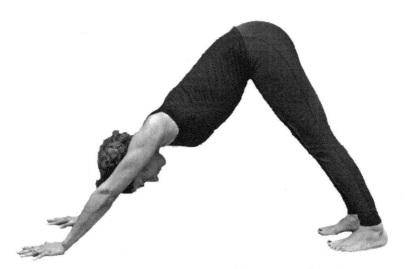

Downward Facing Dog

• Feel you thighs move back engaging your quadriceps.

• Pull your navel towards your spine.

• Tilt your tailbone up.

• Drop your shoulder blades down your back and bring your elbows in.

• Bring your ears in line with your upper arms. This protects your neck while elongating the spine.

• Your feet should be hip width apart.

Cautions:

If your lower back is hurting intensely or you have pain, numbness, or tingling going down your leg, please visit your doctor immediately. While there may be tightness in the back, particularly in the lumbar region, that pain should be mild and under no circumstances should it radiate to another location below the back.

Contraindications:

Very tight hamstrings can lead to a pulled hamstring. Go very gently if you have tight hamstrings, and allow your body to warm up prior to going deeper into this exercise.

Wrists can also be strained with this pose, so if they are troubling you, press down through the knuckles of your index fingers. Use your whole body to bring the force out of your wrists. Move your thighbones back and engage them along with your core muscles.

Pose 7: Warrior I

Instructions:

1. From High Lunge, exhale and lunge forward with your right foot to create a 90-degree angle at the knee.

2. Spin your left (back) foot to a flat position at a 60-degree angle with your heels in one line.

3. Inhale and bring your hands over your head beside your ears, palms facing one another.

4. Hold for 30–60 seconds.

Position:

- Keep heels in one line.

- Square your hips bringing your right (forward) hip back.

- Engage your tailbone by scooping down and forward.

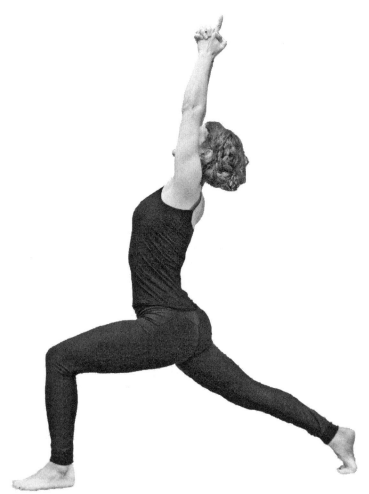

Warrior I

Cautions:

People with high blood pressure or heart conditions may want to consult with a health professional prior to using this pose. If you have shoulder issues, keep arms raised in slightly wider than parallel. If you have a neck problem, do not look up as this can put additional strain on your neck.

Pose 8: Triangle

This is a great pose to stretch and strengthen the thighs, knees, and ankles. It also helps the hips, groin, hamstrings, and calves. Mostly it helps open one's sides up lengthening the spine. It can help relieve sciatica and also backache.

Instructions:

1. Bring your arms parallel to the floor and reach them out to the sides.

2. To work on the left side, turn your left foot out and bring your right foot to a 90-degree angle.

3. Exhale and lengthen your torso, bringing it over the plane of the right leg and bending from the hip, come over the left leg.

4. Rotate your torso to the left so that both sides are long. Drop your left arm down towards the floor. Your shoulders should stack, and your arms should be perpendicular to the floor.

5. Turn your gaze towards the fingertips of your right hand.

6. Hold the pose for up to 1 minute.

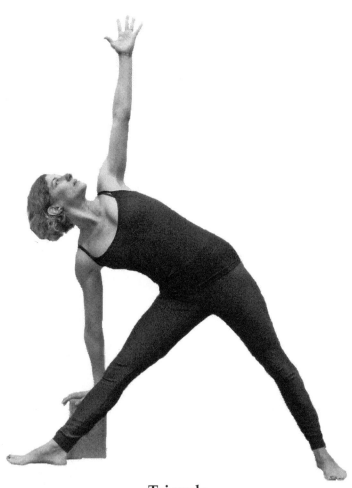

Triangle

Position:

- Keep your palms down and shoulders wide.

- Ensure that the shoulders are stacked and that there is one straight line between the arms and shoulders.

- Keep your heels firmly planted in the ground.

Modifications/Cautions:

- You can use a block on the ground if you can't quite touch the ground.

- If you have neck injury or pain, don't turn your head to look up.

Pose 9: Pyramid

This pose stretches the spine, shoulders, wrists, hips, and hamstrings. It helps improve posture and sense of balance. It is calming too. Similar to the hamstring stretch in terms of the benefits, the Pyramid pose releases the hamstrings so the hips have greater rotation and flexibility.

Instructions:

1. With your left foot forward in high lunge, move the back leg forward so both legs are straight. Keep the back foot flat on floor with your toes facing forward.

2. Round your spine forward and press your forehead into the forward knee. Press heels into floor.

3. Breathe and hold position for 4–8 breathes.

4. Release by moving back into high lunge.

5. Repeat other side.

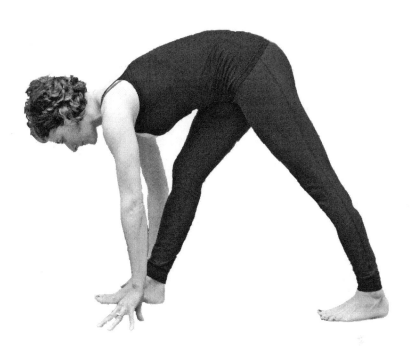

Pyramid

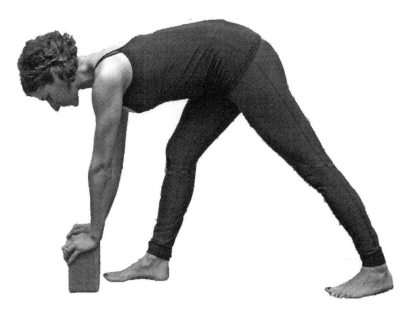

Pyramid Modified

Position:

- Keep your feet on floor.

- Keep the front of your pelvis square to the front.

- Keep your back femur back as far as possible.

- Your front foot should point forward and your back foot will be at a 45–60 degrees.

- Your heels should be aligned in a straight line.

Modifications/Cautions:

- You can practice this with your back heel pressed towards a wall.

- Be wary of recent or chronic injury to the hips, back, or shoulders.

- If you have high blood pressure, avoid the full forward bend. You can do the same thing, but press against a wall without touching your head towards your knee.

Pose 10: Downward Facing Dog

Instructions:

1. From Child's pose, place your hands to the floor about shoulder width apart.

2. Start curling your toes back under your feet and press into the floor.

3. As you press with your toes, press with your hands and start walking your feet toward the back of the mat. Use your hips to lift your body. Keep your knees well bent.

4. Tilt your sit bones up to lengthen your spine.

5. Press down further attempting to place your heels to mat as well, although most people cannot do this.

6. Breathe deeply and freely.

7. Hold the pose for 3–6 breaths.

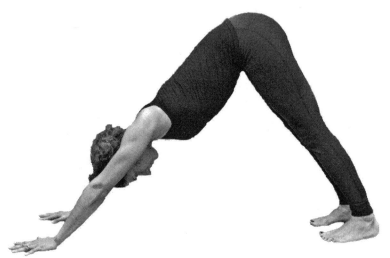

Downward Facing Dog

Position:

- Palms should be flat on the floor and fingers spread apart.

- Feel you thighs move back engaging your quadriceps.

- Pull your navel towards your spine.

- Tilt your tailbone up.

- Drop your shoulder blades down your back and bring your elbows in.

- Bring your ears in line with your upper arms. This protects your neck while elongating the spine.

- Your feet should be hip width apart.

Cautions:

If your lower back is hurting intensely or you have pain, numbness, or tingling going down your leg, please visit your doctor immediately. While there may be tightness in the back, particularly in the lumbar region, that pain should be mild and under no circumstances should it radiate to another location below the back.

Contraindications:

Very tight hamstrings can lead to a pulled hamstring. Go very gently if you have tight hamstrings and allow your body to warm up prior to going deeper into this exercise.

Wrists can also be strained with this pose, so if they are troubling you, press down through the knuckles of your index fingers. Use your whole body to bring the force out of your wrists. Move your thighbones back and engage them along with your core muscles.

Pose 11: High Lunge

Also called the Crescent pose, it helps the lower back and allows for a lengthening of the spine. High lunge is an excellent hip strengthener while stretching the muscles on the opposite side. For golfers, this allows for better range of motion and finish of the golf swing.

Instructions:

1. From Downward Facing Dog, exhale and step forward with your right foot between your hands aligning your knee over the heel. The left leg should be long and strong.

2. Inhale and raise the torso upright.

3. Bring your arms wide and raise them over your head with the palms facing one another.

4. Lengthen your tailbone towards the floor, reaching your left heel.

5. Hold for 4–8 breaths.

6. Exhale and release the torso to the right thigh.

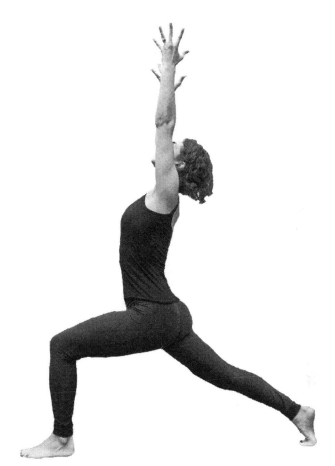

High Lunge

Position:

- Keep your back legs long and strong.

- Arms should be straight over your head with palms facing one another.

- Do not overarch the lower back.

- Bring the shoulder blades deep into the back to support the chest.

- Allow your ribs to drop to the floor.

Cautions:

People with high blood pressure or heart conditions may want to consult with a health professional prior to using this pose. Also it can provoke increased strain in the lower back region.

Pose 12: Standing Straddle Bend

This pose is very good for stretching and strengthening the inner and back legs. It helps relieve mild backache and can also calm one's brain. For golfers, this is a great stretch for the lower back and areas that rotate during one's swing.

Instructions:

1. From Mountain pose, spread your legs about 3-4 feet apart. Taller people will need to keep their legs further apart.

2. Place your hands on your hips keeping your feet parallel to each other.

3. Draw your ankles up, lifting the inner arches of your feet. Press the outer edges of your feet and plant your big toe into the floor.

4. Engage your thigh muscles and lift your chest.

5. Exhale and lean forward from your hips. Place your fingers on the floor directly below your shoulders.

6. Extend your elbows fully.

7. Push your thighs back and continue to lengthen your torso. Rotate the inner groins away from each other.

8. Bend your elbows and lower your torso towards the floor keeping it as long as possible. If you are able, rest the top of your head on the floor.

9. Stay in the pose for about 1 minute. Lift yourself up from inhale and walk yourself back to
   Mountain pose.

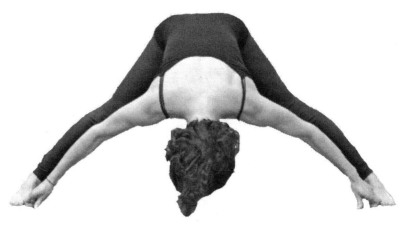

Standing Straddle Bend

Position:

- Keep your arms loose.

- Keep your torso as long as possible.

- If you are doing the modification, keep your arms
  straight behind you.

Modifications/Cautions:

- A block or folded blanket can be placed underneath where the head will touch the floor to make
  it easier for beginning students.

- To intensify the stretch and open the chest, one
  can interlock one's hands behind one's back pri-
  or to bending forward. Be careful to allow the
  shoulders to relax.

- If you have lower back problems, consult with a
  healthcare provider prior to trying this position.

Pose 13: Tree

The pose improves balance, stretches groins and inner thighs, chest and shoulders. It strengthens the thighs, calves, ankles, and spine. This and the next two poses should be done in order on one side and then repeated on the other. The less you can touch your active foot to the ground the better, as this helps to improve balance. For golfers, this pose is extremely important. One of the biggest problems for golfers is a loss of balance. Usually this occurs because one swings harder than their hips will allow. Increasing balance allows one to swing harder and will increase distance of the ball.

Instructions:

1. From the Mountain pose, raise your right heal high and place the sole of your right foot onto the sole of your right foot to your inner left thigh.

2. Press through the sole of your left foot to root into the floor.

3. Keep your hips even. You will need to drop your right hip to do so.

4. Lengthen your tailbone towards the floor. Press your hands together in a prayer position.

5. Stay in this position for 30–60 seconds.

Position:

- Your pelvis center should be directly over your upper foot.

- Keep your hips even.

- Use your abdominal muscles to hold the position.

- Squeeze your elbows in towards each other.

Modifications/Cautions:

- You could use a wall to balance yourself.

- If you feel steady enough, bring your hands above your head.

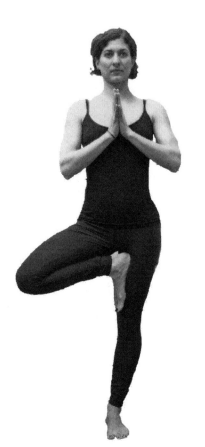

Tree

Pose 14: Eagle

This pose is excellent for improving balance and building lower body strength. It requires concentration and coordination, and it also opens the shoulders and the hips. Eagle is another pose that helps increase balance so that one can swing faster.

Instructions:

1. From a standing position with both arms raised, exhale and wrap your left arm under your right with elbows bent, bringing palms together and thumbs crossed.

2. Exhale and bend your knees to squat. Shift your weight to the right side.

3. Inhale and lift the left leg so that it is crossing over the right knee and wrapping it around the right leg. The left toes should be behind the right ankle.

4. Stare to one point on the wall for balance.

5. Press the shoulders back to keep from leaning forward.

6. Hold for 3–6 breaths.

7. Release by inhaling and uncrossing the arms and legs.

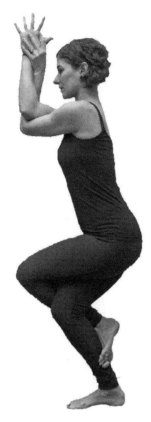

Eagle

Position:

• Keep the thumbs crossed over one another.

• Make sure that the unweighted leg is wrapped in front of the other. The toes should be behind the ankle.

• Staring at a single point allows one to maintain balance.

• The deeper you bend your knee the more stress you may have on the knee. You can relieve that stress by standing taller, although that will work the quads less.

Cautions:

Recent or chronic injury to the knees, hips, arms, or shoulders.

Pose 15: Dancer's Pose

This pose stretches the thighs, groins, and abdomen and also the chest and shoulders. It allows for strengthening of the legs and ankles. Mostly it improves balance. This pose works muscles that improve balance and allows one to swing with more speed.

Instructions:

1. From Mountain pose (or the previous pose), shift your weight to the right foot and lift your left heel towards your buttock bending your knee.

2. Grab your left foot with your left hand pulling your heel into your buttock. Your knee will be pointing straight down. To avoid compression in your lower back, actively lift your pubis toward your navel, and at the same time, press your tailbone toward the floor.

3. Bring your right arm up to the sky and hold for 20–30 seconds.

4. Now lift your left foot up and away from the floor and away from your torso. Extend the thigh back so that it is parallel to the floor.

5. Stretch your right arm forward parallel to the floor.

6. Stay in the pose for 30–45 seconds.

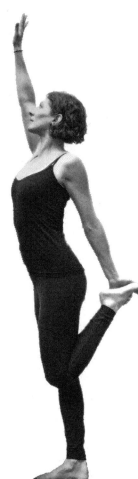

Position:

- Keep your standing leg straight.

- Keep your active arm and active leg parallel to the floor.

- Remember to breathe as you lift your chest.

Modifications/Cautions:

Some beginner's get cramps in the back of their thigh when first attempting this pose. Draw the top of the foot towards the shin to help alleviate this.

Dancer Start

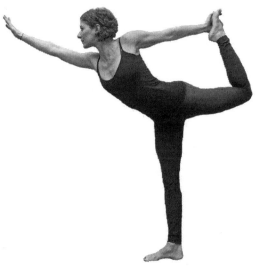

Dancer Full

Pose 16: Mountain

Instructions:

1. Start by standing up straight. Drive your legs down while at the same time lifting your sternum up towards the ceiling. Imagine that you are stretching your feet and your head away from each other. Leave your hands down by your side, as if you are standing at attention.

2. Spin you palms outward, inhale and sweep your hands up sideways stopping when a shoulder's width apart above your head.

3. Lift your chin and gaze up at the ceiling.

4. Hold for 3–5 breaths.

Position:

- Reach your fingertips to the ceiling and root your feet into the floor.

- Keep your eyes focused on one point.

- Pull your stomach into your spine.

Cautions:

There are none for this pose.

There are three sets of sequences and
match if that is your style. Remember to
minimum of 15 minutes a day for 3 wee

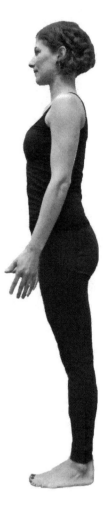

Mountain

Chapter Summary

- Yoga postures can help you gain balance, strength and improve cardiovascular fitness.

- Each pose can be done in sequence to help lengthen and strengthen the body.

- Don't over stretch or try too much at first, but do keep the habit of yoga going to maintain proper alignment.

Chapter 6

Beyond the Course: When To Get Professional Help

You now have a great basis to start working out, learning breath control, diet, and relaxation to start improving your game. At some point though you may need help. Maybe you are having trouble doing a particular pose, or maybe you have more dietary questions. Obviously, there could be other factors that are preventing your game from improving that are related specifically to golf. In those cases, find a golf pro and take lessons. But from learning about health there may be things that are confusing you. In this chapter, the issues of when to see the doctor immediately is discussed and also what we do at our clinic. There are many ways that one can be helped, and this gives a brief overview of some of the types of intervention that can be offered.

Precautions: When to see the doctor?

Probably the most important thing to understand is when to see the doctor. Playing a sport can lead to injuries. Over 50% of all golfers have some sort of injury at one time or another and 40% have chronic injuries. Proper intervention early can prevent an acute injury from becoming a chronic problem. But do you need to intervene every time? There is no simple answer for this. Sometimes, there is nothing that should be done. The body will resolve the situation and healing will occur. For example, we've had several people twist their ankles and other than ice packs and staying off of it, no other medical intervention was necessary for proper healing. The body, when appropriately aligned, rested, fed, hydrated, and with a calm mental state, can heal most conditions. But how do you know if your injury is not more serious? If you do hurt yourself, R.I.C.E. therapy is the best approach within the first 48 hours.

Rest: take a break. Rest the part of the body that is injured.

Ice: Apply an ice pack over the sore area for a minimum of 20 minutes, 3 times a day.

Compression: Use a compression type bandage to reduce swelling. Elastic bandages can be wrapped around the area.

Elevation: If the part of the body is a foot or ankle, raising that body part is very effective in the healing process.

Other times though, you may require a more serious intervention. Here are a few guidelines of when to get further evaluation. These aren't the only reasons you may need to go to the doctor, but these are some of the more common ones.

1. The pain hasn't gone away after a few weeks.

People get pain at times; that is a normal part of exercise. In many cases, one can have pain after stretching or strengthening muscles. Maybe you are engaging muscles that you haven't used since you were a toddler. Generally, this type of pain is short lived and will be gone in a couple of days. Many of my patients experience this type of pain when they first start exercising again. The pain doesn't last long and is a reminder that you have used this muscle and it should be rested.

On the other hand, if you have pain that lasts for several weeks, this is likely affecting your performance. For most people, chronic pain increases stress, which leads to disturbances in blood sugar, mood, and sleep. Some people don't even register the pain; the only sign of a problem is sleep issues, weight gain, or extreme fatigue. Once past the acute phase, the body may start responding in a manner that leads to chronic issues.

2. The pain is extending to other parts of the body or is creating numbness or tingling in one or more of your limbs.

Numbness or tingling in the limbs can be very serious. This needs to be checked immediately. In most cases, the problem is easily treated but there could be a more serious problem arising. There may be a slipped or herniated vertebra, nerve impingement, or other issue that really needs to be evaluated by a medical professional.

3. You get dizzy or faint when doing the exercises.

Dizziness during exercise can be nothing. It sometimes occurs because you haven't eaten, you moved too quickly, or you're fatigued. On the other hand, there could be a very serious issue arising. One could be having blood pressure problems, blood sugar issues, or more serious issues with brain function.

4. You can't slow your mind down enough to meditate or you get very anxious when meditating.

Why is anxiety or not being able to settle one's mind a reason to go to the doctor? It can be a symptom of a physical imbalance. While we live in a society that encourages distraction, we often distract ourselves when uncomfortable. I had one patient who had problems meditating because she was in too much pain to sit still. When sitting she would need to distract herself to not register the pain. In other cases, the patient had imbalances in blood sugar or nutrients that lead to the distraction. Many health professionals will likely want to prescribe medications such as an anti-depressant. In most cases, this is unnecessary and other forms of treatment and work-up are needed.

5. You keep getting sick on this regime.

This particular issue is sometimes difficult to define, as illness may come and go in cycles for a variety of reasons. We have watched people start a new workout regime and run into this problem. There are several reasons for it. Some people have an impaired immunity where they are more susceptible to everything. Other people worked out too hard and lowered their immunity through high cortisol levels. Finally, others were not getting sick so much as releasing toxicity through lungs, digestion, and urination; and while it was uncomfortable, it was a temporary state. Seeing a holistic doctor in this situation can be very effective, as understanding the issue is important to solving it. If it is just that you are eliminating toxins, a good Naturopathic Physician or other holistic practitioner can provide remedies, supplements, and dietary changes that will make this process smoother.

6. You keep injuring yourself.

A common complaint from patients is that they want to exercise, but as soon as they start they get hurt. There can be a lot of things happening here. One is that you may be doing the exercises incorrectly. The other more serious issue is that your body is completely out of alignment and doing the exercise correctly or incorrectly is stressing a weak part of your body. When I first started doing yoga, I ran into this issue because my back was out of alignment. I would do an exercise to stretch my tight groin and I would loosen it only to have it be tighter the next day. I finally realized that my hips were out of alignment, and once they were aligned properly this issue cleared up.

7. You had a fall, accident, or other trauma.

This almost goes without saying, but if you hurt yourself in a fall, go to the doctor. We have treated hundreds of people who had a simple bump that become a more serious issue. Often times a simple bump affects the brain causing problems in seemingly random parts of the body. The problem is that what may be a simple bump to the head could be the last straw in a serious of knocks to the head. Having it followed and tracked is important to getting appropriate care.

8. Sudden onset of sharp pain.

You have sudden onset of pain, pain that comes on immediately when you start a particular pose, or you have redness, swelling, or heat around a sore muscle. Perhaps there's a pain in one of your joints that wasn't there previously.

Any of these situations could mean there is a tear in a muscle, ligament, or tendon. Some patients came in after reporting this and stated that it had been going on for some time but could point to the moment they first felt it. Generally they had torn something. Heat and swelling can also indicate a tear, but they could be the sign of an infection too.

9. You are getting weaker and/or you can't control your bowels anymore.

This situation can be a variety of issues. General weakness could be nothing. It may be that you are more tired than you realized or not sleeping as much as you would need. In some cases, we had people who were actually suffering from sleep apnea. Some people who are starting yoga complain of being weak, but that is a factor of unfamiliarity with the poses. Loss of bowel control though could be an issue with possible nerve damage, spinal problem, or other issue. A healthcare provider will be able to assess and determine the best approaches to treatment.

10. Your sleep is disturbed after doing the workout or your sleep is disturbed in general. (Pain keeps you awake.)

Sleep changes can be a fairly serious medical issue. While sometimes people have a bad night or two, it is generally a more serious problem when you are waking every night or having issues falling asleep. Waking frequently to urinate at night could be the sign of a prostate issue in men, or an infection in men and women. Frequently, pain can raise cortisol levels and interfere with one's ability to sleep.

What I Do To Help

Some time ago, my business coach asked me a question. He said, "If a PGA pro wanted to come in and be treated in three days, what could you do?" At first, I was perplexed. I couldn't fathom how the body could heal in that short amount of time. What would it take to allow for body to become rebalanced in three days? This started a new exploration of treatment regime that allows us to do a lot in a short amount of time. Not only are we finding this approach to be successful, but patients love it! It allows us to treat people in areas of the country who would not have access to our combination of modalities without going to 6 or 7 different providers. They love the convenience and know that we are only a phone call away if they need advice, supplement refills, or other interventions that are slower but more long acting. I practice in Portland, Oregon and on the North Shore of Oahu. There are some wonderful golf courses in Portland including Pumpkin Ridge, The Reserve, and Langdon Farms. Oahu possesses some of the greatest courses on the planet including Turtle Bay Resort (two courses) next to my office.

For those of you that can't commit to coming to Oregon or Hawaii for an intensive, I offer telehealth visits. It is described in more detail below.

In the next pages, we explain some of what we do at our clinic as it provides a wonderful context for how you can gain greater health while also improving your golf game. This isn't to say that everyone's golf game will benefit from this regime. There's an old joke where a patient asks a doctor, "Doctor after my operation, will I be able to play violin?" The doctor responds, "Of course." The patient replies, "That's funny, I don't know how to play the violin now." But just like this patient, if you can't play golf (or play very well) you will not suddenly be shooting scratch golf.

Many of you will call or write me asking what you can do to help your health besides what is in the book. Below are some of the types of treatments that we use at our clinic.

Some of these suggestions are reactive healthcare. What I mean by that is that we only do them when there is a problem with the person. Most of what I describe is in this context. We offer solutions to problems that have arisen. But all of these can be done proactively, meaning that you can use these concepts to prevent health problems before they arise.

We combine all of the techniques listed below in a variety of ways depending upon what the patient needs. At the end of this section we describe how this happens and if you wish to come to our clinic for an intensive, our contact information is at the back of the book. We have specific weeks during the year that we have intensives that change from year-to-year. The easiest way to help yourself is through supplementation.

Supplementation

I offer vitamin and mineral packages specific to some of the problems discussed in the book. While supplementation is a huge component of treating chronic pain and injuries, it can also be extremely useful in preventing problems in the future. Supplements may include herbal remedies, vitamins, minerals, food supplements such as protein powder, or some combination of all of these.

Some of my patients ask if supplements are really neces- Some of my patients ask if supplements are really necessary, and the answer is yes. Most people don't get appropriate nutrition and over time that causes depletions of vital nutrients in the body. Nutrients may be used up due to various problems, such as vitamin D being depleted after a brain injury. Due to mineral depletion in our soil, even if we eat properly, we still aren't getting the quantities needed to sustain health. Many conditions such as anxiety, schizophrenia, depression, and Alzheimer's are being tied to vitamin and mineral deficiencies. Please checkout http://askdrgil.com/walsh-protocol for more information.

Starting out, supplementation is extremely important and can help adjust your dietary needs. For example, there is evidence that various conditions may change our food cravings. Parasite infestation, for example, changes what the host desires to eat. Supplementation can change that balance, not only expelling the parasite, but also changing the food cravings to healthy foods. In time, most of our clients require less. They learn to eat better and gain most of their nutrition through proper diet. Some people have specific issues that can be treated through supplementation. Insomnia, anxiety, high stress, low energy, musculoskeletal pain, and other issues can often be solved through proper supplementation. But for people without these problems, supplementation is a proactive solution to keep them or other issues at bay.

Don't buy just any supplement because the quality of the components isn't the same. There is no requirement for third-party testing of supplements and some don't contain what is on the label.

I offer specialized packs for particular problem sets that people can order. Our supplements are high-grade quality and are testing by an independent third party. We have a simple approach that allows people to respond to a questionnaire and we will send out a monthly supplement supply that is customized to your needs. What our clients love about this approach is that they are only taking what they need for their specific situation without overspending on items that their body doesn't need. Again, please look at the back of the book for contact information and how to order specific packages.

Neurofeedback

Neurofeedback is potentially the most potent tool for golfers and athletes of all kinds. There is research from all over the world that demonstrates how effective it can be in helping people with all sorts of conditions including anxiety, stress, sleep disturbances, concentration difficulties, and headaches. Many people after going through neurofeedback feel as if a fog has been lifted because the problems mentioned above are being caused by an imbalance in the brain.

What is neurofeedback? It is a computer-aided process whereby a person can recognize and modify brain patterns. This allows for better control of those patterns so that one can change them. In a typical neurofeedback session, the person will be seated comfortably in front of a screen and have wires attached to her head. He or she will be watching a movie or video game that is played with one's mind for 30-60 minutes. The game allows for a feedback mechanism where the person attached to the wires is being rewarded for following the pattern being presented. Other forms are much faster, such as Low Energy Neurofeedback System (LENS), where a person sits still with their eyes closed and a minute pulse is introduced into the brain that the brain can use to create new patterns.

With LENS, a map is created over the course of one to five sessions depending upon the sensitivity of the patient. The map gives us insight to what is happening in the person's brain, but most importantly it provides a key as to the areas of the brain that are most important to treat and how to approach treatment.

Neurofeedback has multiple effects. Relaxation is a minimum effect of the treatment, but multiple double-blind placebo control studies reveal that changes are happening within brains receiving neurofeedback. Generally, people find that they can relax more easily even after the sessions are complete and can quiet their minds more easily. Concentration, sleep, anxiety levels, executive function, mood, and organizational ability all may improve with effective neurofeedback sessions. For my patients who are golfers, many reported as much as a 5-stroke reduction in their golf scores as a result of neurofeedback interventions alone. One patient in particular broke 80 for the first time in his life at 65 years of age! He attributed it to the neuro-feedback, as he didn't have any other changes in his habits or game. He found his concentration and sleep improved markedly as well.

There are thousands of studies regarding neurofeedback over the last 50 years that show how effective it can be for a variety of conditions including insomnia, concentration, headaches/migraines, ADD/ADHD, and so forth. For the golfer, it can provide great benefits in focus, concentration, and executive function. This will allow for better scoring. Some of my clients will come in for a neurofeedback session prior to a tournament, as they find this regimen improves their scoring.

UNDA Numbered Compounds/Botanical Medicine

Botanical medicine is another modality that we use at our clinic to help patients heal. In the chapter about diet, we discussed inflammation and the body's ability to eliminate toxicity. The body is like a bucket that fills up and then overflows if it can't eliminate fast enough. Botanical medicine in general, and UNDA-numbered compounds in particular, elicit increased elimination. UNDAs are combination formulas designed to work on particular organ systems. Each number works on the body to better eliminate toxins, promote healing, and improve function of that system. In general, when someone has a chronic injury, healing is not occurring due to an imbalance in the body.

UNDAs help the body begin to balance and heal as more toxins are released from the body. From the perspective of the golfer, this reduces the amount of pain one may feel during a round and reduce the risk of injury.

UNDAs have also been used to help people's emotional states. Problems such as anxiety, insomnia, and concentration difficulties can be treated with UNDAs as a calming agent. Oftentimes, toxins get stored in the nervous system creating a disturbance in sleep, mood, or cognitive function. Obviously, any of those problems can affect performance on and off the golf course. With UNDAs, one can gain benefit without the side effects of other types of interventions.

Relaxation and Meditation

As discussed in the chapter on relaxation, there are many approaches to relaxation and countless benefits. I teach relaxation techniques similar to those that are offered in previous chapters.

Counseling

While I have alluded to counseling, it really hasn't been discussed in the context of helping one improve their game. Counseling can be highly effective to golfers. I use various techniques and methodologies to help people overcome obstacles to playing better. For some people that may be anger management. For other people, I help them with cognitive behavioral techniques (CBT) to reduce stress during tournaments. Each person is different and requires different approaches. Our goal isn't to analyze the person but to give them tools to assist them during play.

Body Alignment

Proper alignment is critical to any athlete, and golfers are no exception. If some part of the body is out of alignment, the rest of the body compensates to allow for the eyes to be looking straight. This means that if your hips are twisted slightly to the right, your spine will subtly compensate whereby your neck is twisted slightly to the left. Needless to say this will mess up a golf swing. I have had many patients complain about suddenly hitting the ball to the right (in a right-handed golfer). I quickly discovered that they had something out of alignment in their left hip and with a simple correction, they were hitting the ball straight once again. Most importantly though, my patients had pain relief from this work and were able to enjoy playing and living their lives more.

Many of our patients have monthly or quarterly visits to maintain optimal body alignment. While diet, exercise, and relaxation techniques all help people with alignment, we sometimes need a tune-up to put things back in place. It allows us to minimize future injuries and improper adaptations that arise from one part of the body being misaligned.

Correct Toes/Foot Care

Our feet are the foundation of our mobility, yet they are completely ignored as part of treatment by many providers. Problems can originate in the feet and continue up through the entire body. Plantar fasciitis is very common, as are bunions, bone spurs, and gout. But did you know that tight hamstrings, ankle problems, shin splints, and hip misalignment can all originate due to foot problems? I not only evaluate feet but also look deeper at some of the problems created by shoes that may cause future issues.

High heels in particular are dangerous for the alignment of the body because heels change the trajectory of the eyes. Humans are programmed to keep their eyes forward. To maintain proper alignment, our feet must be flat on the floor. Otherwise, some part of the spine adjusts to allow the eyes to look center. Any shoe heel changes the center of gravity for the wearer. Wearing them every so often generally isn't a problem. But over time it can create back strain, hip problems, and neck pain and even issues with balance and weakness.

The other problem with many shoes is that the toe box is too small. Watch a barefoot toddler's feet and you see toes splayed out wide to create increased surface area for better balance. When we wear shoes with a narrow toe box, we begin to lose our ability to use our toes to improve balance. After enough time, we lose the ability to move our toes individually. Correct Toes or other toe-spreading products can help restore the wide spread of the toes and improve balance. I still remember the first time I played golf using the correct toes. I felt so stable in my swing and realized how much I fought my own body to maintain balance with small toe-boxed shoes. Now I wear golf shoes with almost no heel and a wide toe box and feel more stable playing. I also feel an advantage as the soles are thin and I can literally feel the breaks of greens as I walk on them.

Products such as Correct Toes are not needed forever though. I recommend starting only 15 minutes a day with them and work up to wearing them all day. After some time, the need for them diminishes and people feel firmer on their feet. And the other foot problems, plantar fasciitis, shin splints, bunions, and so forth diminish or leave all together.

Dietary Advice

Dietary advice is a very important aspect of our treatment, although not as important as some other holistic providers. I look at each individual because no two people are alike. Fortunately, my experience with autism and other neurological conditions has taught us much about how different types of foods can create problems in various individuals. (This is the main reason why I don't like to give general diet advice.) Each person has dietary advice custom made for his or her particular set of problems and more importantly adjusted over time based on their progress.

Hydrotherapy

Hydrotherapy is an effective treatment that I teach. Alternating hot and cold treatments, hot packs, castor oil packs, and other forms of hydrotherapy are extremely effective for healing chronic and acute injuries. Hydrotherapy refers to any type of therapy that uses water as a source of healing. It not only helps one relax, but induces the parasympathetic response (see the chapter on Relaxation). From a healing perspective, this is helpful for both the long and short-term. Long-term benefits have already been discussed, but short-term it can make many of the other therapies easier and more effective. For example, adjustments go smoother after the muscles around the area are relaxed.

Putting It Together

While we have explored all of the pieces of treatment, you might still ask what can you do for me? Generally, that depends upon the person involved but here is a broad overview of our approach. For some people, they just want small things that can help. They will do the exercises in this book and find that they may need a small boost. For them our supplement program was created. I offer different options for general health, energy boost, muscle and joint difficulties and sleep problems.

For other readers they may require more direct interventions. These readers will wish to consult with a holistic physician to address the issues in a focused or direct manner. I mentioned some of the problems earlier that would likely require intervention from a physician. Some require intensive ongoing treatment while others benefit from telemedicine. While I see people in Hawaii and Portland, many people gain great benefit from telemedicine sessions.

Typically, these begin with patients answering a detailed questionnaire about their health. From this, I already have an idea of what systems are out of balance in the body. Labs may be ordered prior to a session depending upon what was found in the initial review. Labs are generally ordered depending upon the patient's complaints and needs. Imaging is sometimes ordered, but generally the patient has already been imaged and those are reviewed as part of this process.

If neurofeedback is part of the treatment plan there are several options that we recommend including, referral to a provider local to the patient or coming to my location to receive treatment.

Once they learn how to best take care of themselves, they find that golf becomes easier. Through all of these practices, understanding about diet, relief of injuries, and a calmer mind, people find their play improves. It may not occur after the first round, but most people notice that their game improves over the course of a few months. For me, I enjoy seeing people reach optimal health so they can not only improve their golf game, but experience life to the fullest. They really do understand that when you feel well, you play well!

Chapter Summary

- Certain problems that arise may be very serious and can require medical attention for proper evaluation.

- A variety of safe and effective treatments exist for a whole host of conditions and problems. Some can easily be solved with proper supplementation.

- Alignment and posture can affect one's health and one's golf swing.

Conclusion

For many people, the information in this book will be forgotten once the book is put down. Some set of you will persevere through the exercises, dietary advice, and poses. You will find greater balance of mind and body. The aches and pains that followed you through every round will drop off and you will find that your scores improve. There will be a moment of complacency, and in dropping off from the practice you will find that the aches, pains, and mental fog return. You will then know that all the effort you put in previously has really paid off and you will once again find the time to do the practices.

At your fingertips is detailed information about how to better take care of yourself and why you should pursue better health. We have looked at diet and the importance of drinking water, and why drinking water is important to maintaining vital bodily processes and eliminating toxins. Breathing was discussed in great detail and an improved understanding of the methods of proper breathing. You know some yoga poses to help your body and will likely learn more from other books, courses, or videos. Maybe you will even meditate and find a calmer presence.

These practices work, but you must take the time to do them. A habit is formed in three weeks. It takes twenty-one days to get something into your system and continue happening. After twenty-one days of eating well, meditating, and performing yoga poses, you will feel strange on the days that you don't do these exercises. Something will be off, as if you were riding a bike without a helmet. (Assuming you ride a bike with a helmet.) There are other books about each of these topics that will be of interest. Good luck and see you on the links!

If you need to reach me, please feel free to do so through my clinic. You can also email me at info@askdrgil.com. If you are interested in our packages or clinics, please call the number below or check the web page below.

Ask Dr Gil:
http://www.askdrgil.com and
http://www.northshorend.com/feelwellplaywell

503.501.5001

About The Author

Dr. Winkelman, a Naturopathic Physician with a graduate degree in psychology, possesses a unique understanding of how the mind and body interact. Since symptoms are your body's attempt to inform you that there is an imbalance, his goal is to uncover and resolve their underlying cause. Dr. Winkelman's work with athletes, particularly golfers, led him to understand that there were many physical and mental health concepts that could allow for improved performance. Dr. Winkelman achieves this by working in close partnership with his patients using nutritional, herbal, and homeopathic medicines along with neurofeedback to return body and mind to balance and ease.

Besides his focus on holistic mental health, he has experience treating people with head injuries including military veterans and people who have been in motor vehicle accidents. He created iCaduceus: The Clinician's Alternative, the premiere web-based alternative medicine database and has written for various medical journals including Holistic Primary Care. He has presented his approach and findings at many conferences and loves to give presentations on his unique approach.

Dr. Winkelman owns and practices in Portland, Oregon and the North Shore of Oahu in Hawaii. While he isn't a scratch golfer, he is an avid one and tries to play as much as he can. He writes fiction and non-fiction and is the author of the forthcoming series "The Lost Books of Moses".

Acknowledgments

Writing a book is not a solo project. From the outside it looks like it but really it is a team effort. First, I'd like to thank Becki Narli who worked so diligently getting the photos right. She photographed Natalia Policelli who was a delightful model for the yoga poses.

I'd like to thank Debbie O'Byrne for her wonderful cover design and her father Chris O'Byrne for his constructive feedback while editing the book.

I am very grateful to my business coaches Charlie Gilkey and Andy Belanger who in their own ways kicked me in the butt to get things done. This book wouldn't be possible with the mentorship from Dick Thom DDS, ND who has taught me so much about health and wellness.

Finally, I'd like to thank my wife Christie and my kids Eli and Amelia for their patience during the process.

Made in United States
Orlando, FL
17 June 2023

34267737R00141